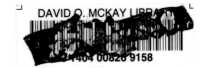

DATE DUE

DEC 1 1 2007		
MAR 0 3 2009		
OCT 1 0 2011		
		Demco

D1505577

Shattered Dreams?

Shattered Dreams?

An Oral History of the
South African AIDS Epidemic

Gerald M. Oppenheimer
Ronald Bayer

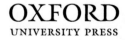

OXFORD
UNIVERSITY PRESS

2007

OXFORD

UNIVERSITY PRESS

Oxford University Press, Inc., publishes works that further
Oxford University's objective of excellence
in research, scholarship, and education.

Oxford   New York
Auckland   Cape Town   Dar es Salaam   Hong Kong   Karachi
Kuala Lumpur   Madrid   Melbourne   Mexico City   Nairobi
New Delhi   Shanghai   Taipei   Toronto

With offices in
Argentina   Austria   Brazil   Chile   Czech Republic   France   Greece
Guatemala   Hungary   Italy   Japan   Poland   Portugal   Singapore
South Korea   Switzerland   Thailand   Turkey   Ukraine   Vietnam

Published by Oxford University Press, Inc.
198 Madison Avenue, New York, New York 10016

www.oup.com

Oxford is a registered trademark of Oxford University Press

Library of Congress Cataloging-in-Publication Data
Oppenheimer, Gerald M.
Shattered dreams? : an oral history of the South African AIDS epidemic /
Gerald M. Oppenheimer and Ronald Bayer.
    p. ; cm.
Includes index.
ISBN 978-0-19-530730-6
1. AIDS (Disease)—South Africa—History.   2. Oral history—South Africa.
I. Bayer, Ronald.   II. Title. [DNLM: 1. Acquired Immunodeficiency Syndrome—
history—South Africa—Interview.   2. Acquired Immunodeficiency Syndrome—
history—South Africa—Personal Narratives.   3. HIV Infections—history—South Africa—
Interview.   4. HIV Infections—history—South Africa—Personal Narratives.   5. Disease Outbreaks—
history—South Africa—Interview.   6. Disease Outbreaks—history—South Africa—Personal Narratives.
7.   History, 20th Century—South Africa—Interview.   8. History, 20th Century—South Africa—
Personal Narratives.   9. Nurses—South Africa—Interview.   10. Nurses—South Africa—
Personal Narratives.   11. Physicians—South Africa—Interview.   12. Physicians—
South Africa—Personal Narratives. WC 503 O62s 2007]
RA643.86.S6S534 2007
614.5'9939200968—dc22   2006033303

9 8 7 6 5 4 3 2 1

Printed in the United States of America
on acid-free paper

To Mathilde Krim, Zena Stein, and Mervyn Susser for their enduring belief in science and their deep commitment to human rights and the global struggle against AIDS

ACKNOWLEDGMENTS

This book would not have been possible without the extraordinary generosity of the doctors and nurses to whom we turned in South Africa. In making time to tell us their stories and in opening up their worlds of work, they provided us with an unparalleled chance to learn about HIV/AIDS in South Africa. To their number, we were able to add a small number of AIDS activists, who allowed us to understand the thread of AIDS-related protests going back to the 1980s.

A project like this also takes financial support. We began with generous gifts from the American Foundation for AIDS Research and the John M. Lloyd Foundation. In addition, one of us (RB) received support from the NIMH-funded HIV Center for Clinical and Behavioral Studies at the New York State Psychiatric Institute. When it was crucial, funding also came from the Rockefeller Foundation and the National Library of Medicine of the National Institutes of Health. Finally, we were privileged to spend a month in the summer of 2005 at the Rockefeller Foundation's Study and Conference Center in Bellagio, Italy, where, in the most splendid setting, we were able to devote ourselves to writing a substantial part of our manuscript.

To write this book required the support of many colleagues and friends. For assisting us in identifying the doctors and nurses we interviewed, we want to thank Alan Berkman, Gerald Friedland, Quarraisha and Salim Abdool Karim, and members of the Southern African HIV Clinicians Society. Robert Sember at Columbia University and Philippe Denis at the University of KwaZulu-Natal in Pietermaritzburg were both extremely helpful in answering questions about South African politics and society. For carefully reading our manuscript and providing sage advice, we gratefully acknowledge Tessa Marcus and Shula Marks. And to our wives, Anne Stone and Jane Alexander, we owe many thanks for their support as we labored on this book.

Finally, we must thank NiTanya Nedd, who masterfully managed our complex travel and interview schedule and became the keeper of our tapes, and Lela Cooper, who demonstrated, as she has in the past, that transcribing taped interviews is both a skill and an art. Last, we want to acknowledge the extraordinary work of Alison Bateman-House, whose intelligence, knowledge, and managerial skills informed every step of our manuscript preparation as we brought this book to a conclusion.

CONTENTS

Shattered Dreams?

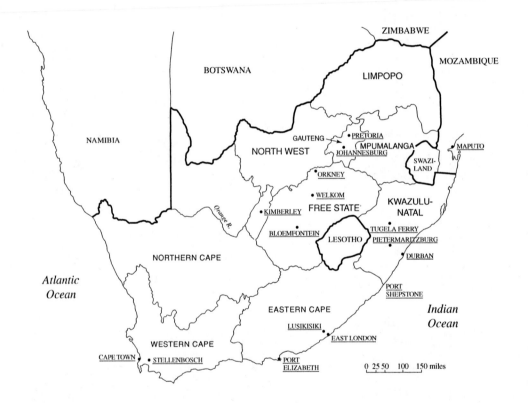

Provincial Map of South Africa with Interview Sites

Introduction

AIDS and the Legacies of Apartheid

On April 27, 1994, the people of South Africa voted in their first democratic, racially inclusive election, thus bringing down the final curtain on 46 years of apartheid rule. Decades of bitter struggle against a racist and oppressive regime had ended. The Soweto uprising of 1976—which sparked widespread protest by students against the government's efforts to impose Afrikaans as the language of school instruction—rent, school, and bus boycotts; militant Black unionism and labor strikes and violence in the Black townships that brought some to the brink of anarchy had been striking manifestations of intensifying opposition. Each expression of protest drew from the government increasingly harsh repressive measures—the occupation of townships by the South African Defense Force, mass arrests, police violence, the torture and assassination of political opponents—as the regime sought unsuccessfully to regain the upper hand. The chaos and repression evoked intense international pressure for reform and disinvestment. Internally, the state suffered from economic stagnation, chronic inflation, and growing white disaffection.[1]

In the end, the African National Congress (ANC), the largest anti-apartheid force, and its allies had emerged victorious. Its leader, Nelson Mandela, released from confinement in 1990 after 27 years of harsh imprisonment, assumed the role of president of a new South Africa.[2] It was a moment of enormous hope. The world bore witness to an expression of democratic aspiration rivaled only by the transformations that shook Eastern Europe and the Soviet Union in the last decades of the twentieth century. But, at the very moment of transition, the seeds of a grave epidemic had already been sown. AIDS has indelibly marked the years since apartheid's end, burdening South Africa's Black community, which had so recently shed the political and social oppression of the old regime.

AIDS did not come as a surprise to the new government. By the late 1980s, epidemiologists, aware of AIDS in South Africa's white gay population and of

3

its toll among heterosexuals in other African nations, had begun to warn of
the prospect of a virulent HIV epidemic. In April 1990, in Maputo, Mozambique,
the International Conference on Health in Southern Africa—cosponsored by the
health secretariat of the ANC, the anti-apartheid South African National Medical and Dental Association, and the Committee for Health in Southern Africa
(CHISA), organized by activists abroad—expressed a deep concern about the
prospects of a South African HIV epidemic, even though the official case count then
stood at less than 500. In a statement that reflected the influence of CHISA
members, the gravity of the situation was made clear. The fault lay with the ruling
National Party:

> The campaign waged by the state has been grossly inadequate. Commu-
> nities have not been consulted. Too little funds have been allocated to HIV
> prevention and the care of people with HIV disease. The media and edu-
> cation campaigns have promoted fear, stigmatization and discrimination.[3]

While a small window of opportunity existed, "the conference agreed that if no significant intervention is made within the next months, there would be little chance of
avoiding disastrous consequences."[4]

The potential severity of the epidemic was understood by some at the highest
levels of the ANC. Chris Hani, the former commander of its military wing, Um-
khonto we Sizwe, and general secretary of the Communist Party, a staunch ally in
the underground struggle against apartheid, warned his comrades: "We have a
noble task ahead of us—reconstruction of our country. We cannot afford to allow
the AIDS epidemic to ruin the realization of our dreams."[5]

So critical was the issue of AIDS that the ANC health secretariat signaled its
willingness to hold discussions with the government's Department of National
Health and Population Development to devise strategies for dealing with the unfolding threat. It was out of these efforts that the National AIDS Convention of
South Africa (NACOSA) was born. In the fall of 1992, a period of considerable
tension and much political uncertainty, it convened a conference—South Africa
United against AIDS—with the goal of developing a national AIDS program. And
so the efforts to confront AIDS, through a broad consultative process involving civil
society institutions, occurred at the very moment that the transition to democratic
rule was taking place. In July 1994, three months after the national elections,
NACOSA issued a National AIDS Plan for South Africa. It spoke in urgent, but
confident, terms about the need to introduce

> effective measures to ensure that this epidemic is contained and the people
> and communities that are infected and affected have care and support. . . .
> The plan proposes a set of interventions which constitute the minimum
> level of such an effective response. This plan is feasible and affordable and
> implementation can be initiated immediately.[6]

But despite such apparent commitment, and the zeal attendant upon the transitions to democracy, AIDS took hold in South Africa, mocking the promises and aspirations of those who understood that half measures and procrastination could prove to be both morally and socially ruinous.

When, in 1994, she assumed responsibility in the post-apartheid Ministry of Health for overseeing the implementation of the National AIDS Plan, Quarraisha Abdool Karim, a 34-year-old microbiologist and anti-apartheid and AIDS activist, quickly became aware that she was saddled by an incompetent, even ignorant, staff composed of individuals held over from the old regime. She told a national meeting of the National AIDS Convention that "the NACOSA plan can't be implemented as is; the budget that we need is not there; the capacity to deliver is not there. We need to look at what each of the sectors can actually do."

A decade later, grim and almost mind-numbing statistics revealed the depths of the failure and the extent of the toll that HIV had exacted. An estimated 5.5 million men, women, and children were infected.[7] More than 500,000 had acquired HIV infection in 2004 alone.[8] Among childbearing women, almost 20 percent were infected, a sevenfold increase since 1991.[9] In the most severely affected province of KwaZulu-Natal, 4 out of 10 women giving birth tested positive for HIV. In 2004, 300,000 deaths were attributed to AIDS, over 40 percent of the mortality in South Africa for the year. The death rate for women 20–39 years of age was more than three times higher than it had been seven years earlier. For men 30–44 years of age, the death rate had more than doubled.[10] Almost 2 million had succumbed since the onset of the epidemic.[11]

Creating an Oral History

The saga of AIDS in South Africa is framed by the increasingly obvious failure to prevent the spread of HIV, first in the gay and then in the Black populations, and to stem the rising tide of death and suffering. This was so even as new, effective therapies began to transform AIDS into a manageable chronic condition in economically advanced nations. Central to this narrative are the struggles of treatment activists in South Africa, beginning in the late 1990s, to make the price of those anti-AIDS drugs affordable;[12] the unexpected and inexplicable decision of President Thabo Mbeki, Nelson Mandela's successor, to embrace theories that challenged the science of HIV/AIDS and his subsequent opposition to the provision of antiretroviral therapy to patients dependent upon the public health care system;[13] and, finally, the remarkable efforts and ultimate success of the grassroots Treatment Action Campaign, led by critics from within the ANC, to compel a reversal of the government's position.

This history might be recounted in many ways, from many vantage points. We have chosen to tell this story through the eyes of doctors and nurses who felt compelled to provide care under circumstances that would become increasingly desperate. We made this decision based on our experience in the United States, where we had written an oral history of the first generation of doctors to care for patients with AIDS. Our book, *AIDS Doctors*, had captured, in their own words, the experiences of men and women who came to AIDS when it was a fearsome, stigmatized disease, when little could be done for the sick and dying.[14] Only at the very end of our account did the entry of antiretroviral therapy begin to change the picture. The trajectory of this book is not dissimilar though it begins almost a decade later.

We understood, from our earlier work, that a book based on oral histories but bolstered by other sources could provide us with insights not otherwise available. It would allow us to hear about and then re-present the depth of commitment, the fears, the despair, the hopes—realized and dashed—of those who cared for men, women, and children with AIDS. By using oral histories, we would not only offer readers an appreciation of what it has been like to be a caregiver in what has rightfully been called the world's worst AIDS epidemic to date, but also a visceral sense of the human toll that has been exacted, a toll often difficult to grasp even as the brutal statistics that define the scope of the epidemic are recited. This was very much on the mind of Brian Brink, the 52-year-old vice president for medical affairs of the giant Anglo American Corporation, when he spoke to us in 2004. Brink, a pragmatic and diplomatic executive, was also capable of speaking lyrically of South Africa and passionately about the needs of those with HIV.

> I see this epidemic as an extraordinary threat to the population of the country. It is a health catastrophe the likes of which have never been seen before in recorded history. I don't think people in the First World fully appreciate the enormity of the statistics. They talk of millions of people dying, but they don't understand what a million means in this context. They don't understand what a thousand means. A thousand people dying is a disaster. I remember September 11th and watching on TV when the World Trade Center was attacked. The horror—and the thousands—three thousand dead. Look at how we react to 3,000, 5,000, or 10,000 persons we didn't know dying in an instant. That many people are dying almost every day in Africa, and we just let it pass us by. We almost become complacent; we accept that this is inevitable. It just happens. People just don't comprehend what is actually going on. You have actually got to get out there and go into those impoverished areas, those rural areas, and see the people dying and the dependent kids that are left behind.

It is through the accounts of doctors and nurses working in South Africa's great urban centers and its impoverished countryside that our story unfolds. Oral histories require intensive work. Our interviews took place during four extended visits to South Africa stretching from January 2003 through January 2005. Those interviewed were drawn from lists of names recommended by colleagues in the United

States who had worked in South Africa and from AIDS experts in that country, including members of the South African HIV Clinicians Society, established in 1998 as a forum for educating caregivers about the treatment of AIDS. In all, we interviewed 73 doctors and 13 nurses, some more than once. Reflecting the legacy of apartheid's severe limitations on the training of Black doctors, 42 of the physicians we interviewed were white; 15 were Indian; only 16 were Black. Consistent with the opportunity for Blacks in nursing under apartheid, only 3 of our nurses were white.[15] Those we interviewed worked in Johannesburg, Cape Town, and Durban; in townships like Soweto and Khayelitsha; in remote rural communities in KwaZulu-Natal and the Eastern Cape; and in the clinical facilities of one of the largest mine operators in the country, AngloGold. Our goal in identifying those we would interview was not to create a sample that was in any conventional sense statistically representative. Rather, we wanted to find physicians and nurses with varied experiences, those who could reflect on elements that were common in the encounter with AIDS in South Africa, and those who could provide insights into the utterly unique.

From the start, it was our intention to identify these doctors and nurses, with their permission, by name and by place of work. These are real actors struggling against political, economic, and scientific limitations to ameliorate the conditions of real patients burdened by the HIV epidemic. Stripping these clinicians of their identities would have detracted from the historical richness, force, and complexity of the stories they have to tell. In a few instances, in specific contexts, those we interviewed have asked us for personal or professional reasons not to reveal their names, and we have complied.

The worlds from which these doctors and nurses were drawn were profoundly shaped by apartheid. So too was the health care system within which they would come to address the unfolding AIDS epidemic.

Apartheid's Legacies

In South Africa, from the earliest colonial years of the seventeenth century, inequality has consistently rested on racial distinctions and the assumption of superiority on the part of European settlers who, with rare exception, held increasing political power over the centuries. Intentional segregation and restrictions on access to resources—economic, educational, and health—on the grounds of color were established facts well before the promulgation of apartheid by the Afrikaner-dominated National Party in the twentieth century. More than a century of inequality had dramatic effects on the Black, Indian, and Colored populations, which experienced higher levels of morbidity and mortality from malnutrition, infectious diseases, occupational disorders, accidents, and violence.[16] Concomitantly, whatever medical services were available were, in the words of the South African physician-ethicist Solly Benatar, "directed mainly by whites for whites, good health, in effect, being deemed more important for whites than non whites, while a long history of insufficient interest in the health status of black patients is discernible."[17]

From 1948, when the National Party came to power, until 1990, when reforms began to dismantle apartheid, life was defined by an official ideology that systematized, justified, and extended racial and ethnic inequality at every level of national and personal life.[18] The National Party codified previous regulations and passed legislation that refined and defined race and interracial relations, using the institutions of the state to enforce rules that affected everyone's life prospects and were the source of humiliations in matters grand and intimate.[19] Influenced by Germanic and Nazi doctrine, the theorists of apartheid—"apartness"—proposed a society in which state-defined racial groups would be coerced or permitted to follow their "inherent" but separate development as "peoples." People were classified into ethnic and racial categories and compelled to live in segregated, homogeneous enclaves, with social intercourse of any sort between groups held to a minimum and, when necessary, limited to a nexus of service or employer-employee relations. With its control over the media and education, as well as its police powers, the apartheid state was able to keep large portions of its population quiescent for much of the period between 1948 and 1976, when the Soweto uprising occurred.

Looking back on how he believed white South Africans viewed those years, Ruben Sher, who would become one of the first AIDS researchers in the country, said:

> As a white person it was wonderful. We lived in good surroundings, we all made reasonable livings, we owned motor cars, we went on holiday. I think most whites didn't care very much about the lot of the Black people. There was a lot of propaganda about the *swart gevaar*, the Black danger, that around everything there was a communist. Most whites were terribly worried about what was going to happen to us once the Blacks took over. The history of Black Africa was not that marvelous.

The geographic boundaries of the white "nation" coincided with the economically most developed and richest urban areas, arable land, and known mineral deposits. Indians, the majority of whom were descendants of indentured laborers brought to South Africa to work in the sugarcane fields in Natal, and the "Colored" population—people of mixed white, Asian slave, San aboriginal, and African origin—were "separated out" through the Group Areas Act of 1950 to serve as a buffer between whites and Black Africans. The Black African majority, constituting almost 70 percent of the population, were dispossessed of their land and their freedom, while their presence in the towns and cities was regulated by pass laws and rules of settlement that attached them to supposedly indigenous "homelands" or "Bantustans," formerly called "native reserves." These impoverished and grossly overcrowded enclaves were scattered across the country, covering approximately

13 percent of the land. Geographical separation and official ideology served to obscure the plight of Black people, making it possible for whites to ignore the conditions under which the vast majority lived. Salome Charalambous, the child of émigrés from Cyprus, grew up in the 1980s. She recalled her mother's utter disbelief when confronted with the conditions that existed in the Black townships:

> Living in South Africa in the 1980s, you were told a lot of things that were not true. You were brought up in a white society, everybody wealthy and well-off, and you never saw the poor people; you never saw how they struggled. For instance, we used to drive past Soweto and see all the nice houses, because at that time the squatter camps were kept far away from the streets; no one ever got to see the squatter camps. The first time I showed my mother a squatter camp, I said to her, "Ma, do you know that people live there?" She said, "No, how can they live there? They can't live there." "Ma, can you see the people?" "No, I can't see them."
>
> We were indoctrinated to believe that everyone was given a house; they were given electricity and running water; and you drove past the townships and thought that everything was fine. We knew about the township strife, but were told things like, "We build them schools and then they burn them down." We were told that these are just bad people; they don't have any family values, they don't have any culture. That's how we were taught.

Deprived of education beyond that which was required for menial labor ("Bantu education"), legally barred from skilled and professional employment as well as independent entrepreneurial activities, and with insufficient arable soil to feed their families, Blacks were forced to accept low-level jobs in areas designated for whites only—farms, mines, domestic households and urban factories, offices and shops. There, they endured strict regulation of their movement, segregation, police surveillance, nightly curfews, low wages, poor access to public services, long separations from family and kin, and unremitting prejudice, discrimination, and political impotence.

In principle, once unemployed—because of economic downturns, political resistance, illicit acts, illness, or old age—most Blacks lost what was deemed to be their privilege to live and work in white South Africa and were forced to "go home" to their Bantustans. Lying in scattered fragments along the white continuum, according to a contemporary observer, these "functioned as dumping grounds for millions of people who were not 'needed' by the 'white' economy. . . . The social costs of supporting all these economically 'surplus' people [were] thus 'exported' to the Bantustans."[20] There, social services were the least adequate in the country, underfunded by the South African government on which the homeland authorities depended.

The migratory dynamic of Black economic and social life, exacerbated by the separation of family members, had a deep, systematic effect on the majority's physical, psychological, and social health throughout the twentieth century.[21] In a classic paper published in 1949, which might well have served as an introduction to the state of affairs almost a half century later, Sidney Kark, a leading figure in South African social and community medicine, argued that syphilis and other diseases epidemic in the Black population were produced by a constellation of social relationships, including commercial or casual sex and increased male-on-female sexual violence,[22] that emerged from the continual movement of massive numbers of workers. In South Africa, he wrote:

> Very few adult men have not been away from their rural homes to work in some town or other. In a number of areas, the majority of men are away during the course of each year.... All this has been going on at an ever-increasing rate since the diamond digging days, producing great changes in Bantu social customs, breaking down a system of rigid moral standards, destroying the old concepts of right and wrong, cheapening relations between men and women and bringing with it syphilis. Without an understanding of the economic factors involved and the historical development of the vast social pathological changes brought about during the last 70 years, no [individual] treatment will save the spread of syphilis in South Africa.... The first line of treatment must be to remedy the unhealthy social relationships which have emerged as the inevitable results of masses of men leaving their homes every year.[23]

The inequalities borne by Black Africans were reflected in other diseases as well. In adults, gastroenteritis, pneumonia, and tuberculosis were rife.[24] Tammy Meyers, now a pediatrician treating children with AIDS, who like most whites under apartheid grew up ignorant of what life was like for the majority, learned, once in medical school in the mid-1980s, "In the white-only hospitals, you saw diseases of affluence in adults, cardiac disease, infarcts; generally it was diseases of Western countries. And then, when you came out to Black hospitals, it was always diseases of poverty."

Among Black workers, those who labored in the mines have come to symbolize many of the problems faced by those who were not white. Historically, rates of tuberculosis were very high in these migrants, who lived crowded into hostels operated by the companies and whose lungs, pitted with lesions formed by the inhalation of occupationally produced dirt and dust, were more susceptible to infection. Before the 1980s, Black miners suffering from active tuberculosis were, like others suffering from debilitating diseases, "repatriated" to their homes within and beyond South Africa's borders, where they could seed the disease in the community before dying themselves.[25] Beginning in the late 1940s, tubercular miners, although undergoing the new TB chemotherapy, rarely received a full course of treatment, because they were repatriated after two weeks to three months,[26] raising a new danger: increased levels of drug-resistant bacteria.

In 1990, there were 183 cases of tuberculosis per 100,000 population reported in Blacks, but only 16.5 in whites.[27] Such stark evidence understated the disparities that prevailed. As the apartheid regime gave ten homelands "independent" or "self-governing political status," with their own governments and health services, the high disease rates suffered by their "citizens," previously part of South Africa's statistics, were now credited to these Bantustans. Umesh Lalloo, a pulmonologist at Durban's previously Black-only hospital, King Edward VIII, and a leader of the anti-apartheid National Medical and Dental Association (NAMDA), noted that in the early 1980s:

Half the patients we used to admit had TB. We were always witnessing and being involved in the TB epidemic. At the time, it was not acknowledged by government because of the way statistics were collected. The patients, many of them who developed TB, came from a section of Natal which was a quasi-independent state, so it didn't feature in the Durban City Council statistics. But if you worked in a Black hospital, you were well aware of a major TB epidemic. In the early 1980s, we used to see patients with advanced TB, TB with extreme poverty, who looked no different than patients with advanced AIDS today.

Infants and children were especially vulnerable. Between 1980 and 1985, for example, infant mortality per 1,000 births carried away 82 Black African babies under the age of one, a rate more than four times that which prevailed among Indians and more than six times that which existed for whites.[28] Deaths of children one to four years of age stood at 2.8 per 1,000 Black Africans, more than three times greater than in the white population (0.8 per 1,000). And malnutrition, to which babies and children were particularly susceptible, was responsible for 9.8 Black or Colored deaths per 100,000 population, almost 25 times higher than the rate among whites (0.4 per 100,000).

Jamila Aboobaker, an Indian-born doctor with ward experience dating to the 1970s and now chief of dermatology at King Edward VIII, South Africa's second-largest hospital, recalled, "We used to see at least three to five babies dying on the day of admission. They came in so bad, with such severe infections and malnutrition that they had no hope. They died before the antibiotics could work." Henry Sunpath, a South African Indian who did his residency training in the impoverished Transkei homeland in the 1980s, recalled the devastation caused by measles: "It was quite sad to see. We lost a lot of children."

Disease and death as distillates of deprivation defined the experience of working in hospitals. Helga Holst, a Canadian-born devout Christian who would, in the context of the AIDS epidemic, work with Henry Sunpath in Durban, looked back on her years of service in a rural ex-missionary hospital and spoke of "stories which still break my heart about juveniles with diabetes who didn't live; and it wasn't because we didn't have insulin. It was because they lived in rural areas, and how do you manage an insulin-dependent diabetic who cannot read or write and can't keep insulin cool?"

Neil McKerrow, a 32-year-old pediatrician completing his specialized training in Cape Town in 1988, near the rich vineyards of Stellenbosch, was stunned by what he saw among the children for whom he cared:

> I didn't pay a lot of attention to the political milieu, but the social cir-
> cumstances of the individual children, which were the consequences of the
> apartheid system, were very obvious. I remember being in touch with
> the Food and Allied Workers' Union, because we would have children
> of factory workers who couldn't afford to feed their kids. We had a
> huge incidence of fetal alcohol syndrome because of the system on the
> wine farms, where workers would be paid in aliquots of wine instead of
> wages.

Institutionalizing Inequality

In modern societies, the health care system, responsible for saving lives and staving off disease and mortality, serves as a rich expression of who is valued, who is considered dispensable. Among the sick, what medical interventions will be available? Who will be excluded, left to suffer illness, pain, and death, to endure psychological privations, when others are not?

Apartheid medicine vividly reflected how differently the worth of Black and white lives was calibrated. Particularly after 1960, the government fostered and extended a dual health care system. A fee-for-service private market became increasingly available to whites with health insurance—sponsored voluntarily by their employers. Many whites, however, and the vast majority of the Black population depended on publicly supported hospitals and clinics. The private system offered medical care comparable to that found in developed countries. But even within the public system there were gross inequalities; whites were assured the newest and best-equipped and -staffed facilities.[29]

In the mid-1980s, the number of beds in Black hospitals and wards per 1,000 individuals was half of what was available for whites (4.2 versus 8.2 per 1,000). In the Black homelands, the differences were even greater; the bed ratio for Blacks was one-quarter of that for whites in South Africa.[30] With the number of Black patients generally outstripping the supply of hospital beds, hospital superintendents used all available space. Typically, as Umesh Lalloo, then a young doctor, described it, "For every patient on a bed at King Edward VIII in the 1980s, we had another under the bed. It's a pity we missed the opportunity to photograph all of that, but we took it for granted; that's the way we were trained." In Pietermaritzburg, at Edendale, according to McKerrow:

There was one ward; the back half was just cots, cheek to jowl, with two or three children per cot. Their nappies, or diapers, would be changed three times a day; so if they soiled their nappies after they had just been put on, they stayed in those nappies for hours. Come meal times, the nurse would sit in front of the cot and feed three children with the same spatula from one bowl.

And at Baragwanath, now Chris Hani Baragwanath Hospital,[31] which served the vast Black township of Soweto, abutting Johannesburg, so little money was invested in the 1980s and so crowded were conditions that, according to Haroon Saloojee, a neonatologist, "Doctors took the extreme measure of writing a letter of complaint, which 100 doctors signed; the conditions for patients were inhumane. The government response was very severe, because it fired all 100 doctors."

Where they existed, the wards and wings assigned to Blacks were starkly inferior to those available to whites, although not necessarily worse than the public facilities meant for Indian or Colored patients. Because medical schools used public hospitals to train students, many doctors had vivid memories of them, recalling how overcrowded the wards and clinics were. Jerry Coovadia, who went to India in 1959 for his medical training and who would become chair of pediatrics at the Nelson R. Mandela School of Medicine, bluntly described what King Edward VIII was like under apartheid: "The services were pretty awful, but the worst I can think of was the neonatal nursery. It was an absolute black hole of Calcutta, a tiny place filled with newborn babies, exactly the environment which will spread infectious disease and make proper care impossible."

Maternity services in the institutions designated for Blacks, Indians, and Coloreds were primitive, providing minimal space and comfort. Neil McKerrow recalled that at Edendale, the Black public hospital in the provincial city of Pietermaritzburg, northwest of Durban, "In the labor wards, you could walk down the passage, very little space between the beds, no curtains, and see every single woman delivering her baby, with no privacy and no consideration for the emotional needs of the patients." Contrasting Edendale with Grey's, the white public hospital, each characterized by long central corridors, McKerrow said, "If you twisted or broke your ankle and fell down in the passage at Grey's, you would probably starve to death, because the number of people in the hospital was pretty small; if the same thing happened at Edendale, you would be trampled to death within five minutes."

Crowding was accompanied by great disparities in technical resources. Bongani Thembela, born in 1958 and one of the relatively small number of Black doctors trained under apartheid—in 1980 they constituted less than 2 percent of the total[32]—recalled conditions at King Edward VIII in 1983, the year he completed medical school: "It was supposed to be the main teaching hospital for the University of Natal, but we didn't have a brain scan, although Addington, which was a satellite, mainly white hospital, had one. Hospitals servicing largely African people were underresourced at the time."

Conditions in rural areas were even worse. Only 5 percent of South Africa's doctors practiced full or part time in the Black homelands in 1962, a proportion that fell to just over 4 percent in 1974 and 3 percent in the early 1980s, even as the population grew.[33] Nurses often provided services where doctors were absent in these settings. But nurse-to-population ratios were also increasingly unfavorable.[34]

Tony Moll, a Christian doctor, came to the Church of Scotland Hospital in impoverished Tugela Ferry in the mid-1980s, more than a decade after the apartheid state had nationalized the approximately 100 missionary hospitals which, with international support, had traditionally offered health care in the home-lands.

In 1986, when I arrived, I was one of five doctors working in the hospital, struggling with very basic things like telephone communication, water supply, laboratory equipment; medication wasn't a problem. We did what we could with limited resources. We would not have a lot of laboratory access. In those days, if I had to find an appointment with a surgeon, it could take a full week. In those days, it would take three or four hours to arrange for an ambulance; the ambulance would be somebody's pickup, and basically hanging the [IV] drip on the back of the van.

Glenda Gray, a pediatrician who, as the child of a communist, anti-apartheid engineer working in the mines, dreamed in her youth of the coming revolution, chose to spend part of her training at Natalspruit Hospital in the then-Transvaal, now Gauteng Province, rather than in the white institutions available to her in Johannesburg. Her memory of what she confronted was particularly graphic:

The further you got out of Johannesburg, the worse it became, and where I did my obstetrics was horrendous because it was a kind of secondary-level obstetrical care. There was poor supervision of the women in labor, poor access to intravenous drips, poor access to pain control, not well-supervised deliveries; women would have cesarean sections when their babies were just about moribund. A lot of birth asphyxia, which means that people weren't taken care of in labor. The facilities were horrible, depressing. They were run by poorly qualified doctors who didn't really care. You would phone them, and they weren't available. You would find your-self as a student having to make decisions, and the baby is being born dead, the kind of thing which you would never, ever see maybe at Bar-agwanath Hospital, and you definitely wouldn't see at the Johannesburg General, then an all-white facility.

The segregation of the public hospitals, which persisted in many places until the early 1990s, was breached at times, although not openly. Andrew Ross, who had come to South Africa in 1975 as a 14-year-old, described how the rules might be bent, even by those who unreservedly supported the apartheid regime:

> I went to a place called Bethel Hospital. It was just outside Johannesburg in a small, conservative town, predominantly Afrikaner people who voted for the National Party. And the doctors you came across really believed that the national government was doing a good job, and that racial segregation was good for the country. It was a "properly" constructed hospital. On the white side, there were smaller, more personal wards; on the Black side there were prefab buildings. There was a time during the year when the operating theater on the Black side was closed. It wasn't seen as acceptable to wheel patients from the Black side through the white side to the theater. So what they would do, they would load Black patients in an ambulance, and they would drive them all the way around the block, so that they could come in through the back door of the white theater. I hadn't seen this before; I hadn't realized that these were the kinds of realities for many people in South Africa.

Kathryn Mngadi, a 24-year-old Colored doctor, served her internship at Addington Hospital in Durban, a predominantly white facility with an old wing for Colored patients. People of other races could be admitted provisionally, a condition that allowed Mngadi, who had been involved in anti-apartheid demonstrations while in medical school, to elude institutional strictures:

> Back in 1988, we were only allowed to admit Indian or Black patients if it was an emergency. So if someone came in with severe asthma, we'd stabilize them; but the next day we were meant to transfer them to their own hospitals. I had a consultant; he must have been in his late 60s or early 70s. It was those long old wards where you had two rows and a division and then another row. So I remember we admitted Mr. Naidoo with asthma and stabilized him. And the consultant got to his bed and said, "You must try and get this patient to R. K. Khan" [the Indian hospital]. So, the next day, we moved him a couple of beds down, and when the consultant got to Mr. Naidoo, he said the same thing. But he never realized, in the man's two weeks of stay, that it was the same man!

Experiencing Inequality

The segregation of hospitals applied not only to patients, but to staff as well. Until the 1980s, Black, Indian, and Colored doctors could not treat patients in white hospitals, and in some facilities a color bar precluded them from giving orders to whites.[35] Ramesh Laloo Bhoola, born in 1943, was old enough to recall what these institutions were like in the years before even modest reforms had occurred. With some bitterness, he remembered:

> It might make you laugh, but I couldn't admit my white patients to hospital in Durban. In '76 I had a white patient who had a stroke; he came to me and I admitted him to hospital, and the next day the manager of the hospital called me up and said, "You cannot treat this patient." I asked why, and he said, "You cannot give instruction to the white nurses." So I was asked not to treat, not by the patient, not by his family, but by the manager of the hospital. So the patient was transferred to a white physician.

Among the most vivid and painful memories centered on the rules that prohibited Black, Indian, and Colored doctors from touching white patients or even seeing them disrobed. Before 1981, according to Ashraf Grimwood, a gay Colored doctor who described himself as "a product of 300 years of cross-cultural insemination," students like his own father were not permitted to examine white patients. "Black students were asked to leave when white patients were brought in, and Black patients were allowed to be examined by everybody." Haroon Saloojee, who graduated from Witwatersrand Medical School in 1984, remembered previous generations of doctors "who would not be able to go to postmortems when there were white bodies."

Discrimination extended to training and remuneration as well for both nurses and doctors.[36] Ashraf Grimwood's father had told him, "In tutorial groups, some of the more famous doctors, like Christiaan Barnard, did not turn up if there were Black students in the group." And Saloojee recalled:

> The professors were all at the white Johannesburg Hospital and we would never have rounds with them. The first time we would encounter all the senior professors was in the examination situation. So my education was deprived. I was not being exposed to the key people.

Ramesh Laloo Bhoola, who had trained in Durban because of apartheid era restrictions, remembered the moment when Indian doctors chose to protest such discrimination; the results were both blunt and catastrophic:

> I was an intern when the senior doctors at King Edward were unhappy because the white specialists were paid differently from Indian specialists, and Indian doctors were paid differently. And they were protesting, not holding placards, but having meetings about this. So they were told, "If you don't like the system, then you must leave." So all of them left. They left! But there was no place to work.

When Ashraf Grimwood qualified as a doctor in the early 1990s, he recalled, "I was of the first group of nonwhite medical students to be paid the same rate."

Battling Racial Inequality

Reflecting the increasing willingness to challenge apartheid's institutions, those doctors who saw themselves as a part of the broader struggle for liberation began to confront the embedded racial biases of the medical care system. In 1982, a small group of doctors, mainly Indians associated with the University of Natal's medical school, organized the National Medical and Dental Association with the aim of fighting against the regime and for a nonracial health care system.[37] The NAMDA took it as an article of faith that, in the absence of a nonracist democratic system of government, no just health care system could exist. It fought apartheid by developing a platform of demands that would attract and mobilize progressive doctors: supporting universal, publicly funded, nonsegregated health care; providing medical assistance to the victims of police and army violence; documenting the physical and psychological trauma suffered by detainees; and discrediting the mainstream Medical Association and Dental Association of South Africa—both supporters of the apartheid government. To further its aims, NAMDA worked closely with the banned ANC, the Natal Indian Congress—formed in 1894 by Mahatma Gandhi—and the United Democratic Front, an alliance of over 500 organizations formed in the early 1980s to counter government plans to sow even further racial divisions. Beginning with 52 doctors, NAMDA membership peaked in 1987 at 2,000, embracing approximately 10 percent of all physicians in South Africa at the time.[38]

Clive Evian, who was an anti-apartheid activist and an officer in NAMDA, recalled working with those who had been detained by the government as it struggled to contain the rising tide of opposition:

> I used to see detainees on a regular basis. We would see especially these youngsters, 14, 15, and 16, as they came out of prison. They had been tortured and beaten up or just kept in there. Quite often, they weren't actually that severely physically damaged but very psychologically stressed out, very confused, very posttraumatically stressed. Actually, they wouldn't let them out if they had any sort of torture wounds. They would keep them there until there was no evidence of that. We documented all this.

Workers associated with NAMDA took considerable risks by assisting people caught in the violence within the townships. Quarraisha Abdool Karim, whose political awakening began with the Soweto uprising, remembered the mid-1980s:

> The repression was so extreme that people who had received gunshot injuries, mainly police brutality, if they went to seek care in the hospital, would be arrested. I was part of a group that was doing first aid training. The police and the army would go in, in the middle of the night, into townships and just randomly shoot and loot, and people then couldn't

come out of the township until the morning and seek care, as there wasn't much service within the townships themselves. We started to train large numbers of people within the townships to deal with emergency situations, how to render first aid, how to deal with wounds. Once they had managed that situation, the immediate crisis was, who were "safe" doctors? We had a network of medical practitioners.

As part of the emergent protest movement, Haroon Saloojee, while still at medical school, worked to desegregate the public hospitals. Despite attending Witwatersrand, considered one of the leading liberal universities, he could recall almost no support among white classmates or administrators. "We tried to push an agenda of admitting Blacks to white hospitals and didn't get much support from our white seniors and colleagues." Soon after Saloojee's efforts, a few white students began to press for change as well. Glenda Gray, more radical than most of her peers, recalled, "There was a group of ten. We objected to working in white hospitals until, first of all, Black patients could go into those hospitals and Black students could go into those hospitals."

When desegregation of hospitals did occur, it came in waves, part of the steady pressure building against apartheid. Gray recalled her action at Johannesburg General, the all-white public hospital, and the swift response of its professional staff. Like the collapse of the Berlin wall, the event was exhilarating, public, and seamless, an action for which the time was ripe:

> I can remember when we started desegregating hospitals, how there was an attempt to bring Black patients into white hospital[s]. This happened in 1988. At that stage only special nonwhite patients could go into those hospitals; if they had a kidney problem or a heart problem then the only place they could get care was at the white hospital. Then, when desegregation became official, white parents objected to their children lying next to a Black child. The good thing was that the doctors actually were merciless, and it came down from the heads of departments, so no one tolerated the views of the parents. We just moved Black kids into the wards, and within a week everyone had forgotten they objected. Everybody worried about these things, and when it happened, it was like a non-event.

At other hospitals, the administration was less sympathetic to change, but the results were much the same. In Durban in the early 1990s, Addington Hospital faced a crisis of desegregation. Kathryn Mngadi, who, following her internship, remained there for five years, recalled:

> While I was in the outpatient department, there was a public protest at the fact that the hospitals were segregated. We were called by the management of the hospital. Oddly enough, although I am Colored, I was in the white

outpatients' part of the hospital; so I only saw white patients. People were planning to come to the hospital en masse and demand to be seen at the white section of the hospital. And the management called us. Basically they said, "Look, you're going to have all these people coming. Listen to their stories, their complaints. Don't really bother to treat them. Give them some medicines and just get rid of them." I didn't say much, but when the marchers actually came and demanded to be seen, the odd thing about it was that they were medical students that had been behind me. There were colleagues that had qualified before me, who were actually really sick with minor things, tonsillitis or flu, but they had symptoms and signs. And I remember thinking to myself, "If I had listened to that director I would have found myself in such trouble, and I doubt that the hospital would have stood behind me." I saw the patients that day like I would see any patient who came to me. And, I'm not sure how long after that demonstration it was, but the hospital was opened up to everybody.

As the racial barriers began to crumble, class divisions took on added salience. The continued expansion of the private medical system was fostered by the government's need to curb its rising health care costs and the desire by business interests, including the insurance industry, to move into lucrative areas long dominated by the state.[39] They were more interested in one's ability to pay than in race or ethnicity, transforming, in the words of one South African health care scholar, "the criteria of differentiation, inequality and discrimination from race to class, or from skin color to purchasing power."[40] Consequently, private health care facilities were opened to Black elites and, later, as Black labor organizations bargained for medical benefits, to workers.[41] As resources for an already strapped public health system fell further behind those available in the private sector, it became clear that privatization, so attractive to those who could afford it, would only serve to exacerbate the deep inequalities in a system that would be inherited by the post-apartheid state and that would be called upon to meet the challenge of AIDS.[42]

Changes in the health care system were but part of much broader transformations occurring in South Africa. In February 1990, after ending a state of emergency declared five years earlier, new leadership in the National Party government under F. W. De Klerk "unbanned" its opponents, the African National Congress, the Pan Africanist Congress, and the South African Communist Party. Political prisoners were freed and fundamental apartheid laws were repealed. Even before such actions were taken, the country's largest corporations had begun a dialogue with the ANC with the aim of influencing policies for the inevitable post-apartheid era, concerned especially about moving the party away from its Marxist economic declarations. Ian Sanne, a Johannesburg doctor whose father had headed the local affiliate of Siemens, the German electronics giant, recalled:

My father was involved through the German South African Chamber of Commerce with all the leadership of the ANC already in the later 1980s, before the release of Nelson Mandela. He spent a lot of his time negotiating with the ANC to get the policy of nationalization of businesses off the table and the policy of free-market economy on the table.

The end of the old order was not smooth. In the growing unrest, Black-on-Black violence escalated, often aided and abetted by the government, which provided assistance to rivals of the United Democratic Front and the ANC. Among these, the most important was Inkatha, headed by Chief Mangosuthu Buthelezi, which drew mainly on a rural Zulu base. In KwaZulu and Natal, a virtual civil war raged between supporters of Inkatha and the ANC. As the head of the Department of Medicine at Edendale Hospital in Pietermaritzburg in the late 1980s, James Muller was witness to the bloody strife in the province. In the hopelessness and violence of those days, including the loss of housing, jobs, and lives, he saw the preconditions for the spread of sexually transmitted diseases, including AIDS, in a province which would come to suffer the highest rates of HIV infection in South Africa:

I knew the conditions were right here for the AIDS epidemic to happen, comparable to Uganda and Zaire. We had this low-grade civil war that was going on in KwaZulu-Natal between the two political parties, the Inkatha Freedom Party and the ANC. It disrupted community life terribly, so people didn't have any hope. I am sure there was a lot of sexual activity going on, because people didn't worry about tomorrow. There was no knowing when someone was going to come and shoot you. People just got on with their lives and enjoyed themselves while they could. And a lot of taboos in society broke down.

It is not the least of the ironies of AIDS in South Africa that, in its death throes, the apartheid regime helped fuel an epidemic that would so mar the first decade of freedom.

1

The Forgotten Epidemic

Despite its international pariah status and relative isolation, South Africa saw its first cases of AIDS in the early 1980s, at the same moment that the disease was recognized in the United States and Western Europe. And, like the epidemics of the wealthy industrialized nations, AIDS in South Africa struck gay men first. Racial cleavages engendered by colonialism and apartheid would assure that the epidemic would remain largely confined to gay white men for some time.

With the acceleration of the vast heterosexual epidemic of HIV in South Africa in the 1990s, it was all too easy to forget that AIDS had begun to take its toll on gay men almost a decade earlier and to forget the bitter experiences of those who had come to treat them. Steven Miller, a 49-year-old specialist in private practice, was one of the first gay doctors to treat men with AIDS at Johannesburg Hospital. In 2003 he remarked on how, after Nelson Mandela's election, the seismic political and epidemiological shift produced something akin to amnesia even among the otherwise well informed. "It was easy to draw a line under everything that belonged to the previous ten years." A new political order "almost makes this the beginning of a new era in all aspects of life." For Miller, who had seen hundreds of patients suffer and die, such forgetfulness represented a profound "disservice" to those who had been sick and their lovers, families, and caregivers.

Miller was one of a handful of doctors, most of whom were gay, who treated patients and provided what little medicine could offer in the first years of the AIDS outbreak. It is their accounts that capture the experiences of an epidemic all but lost to public memory.

Doctors who were drawn to the epidemic as AIDS took off in South Africa's Black population unapologetically speak of the epidemic in gay men as if it happened in another world, as well as a different time. For some, it was simply a matter of working in institutions that served only people of color. Farida Amod, a young infectious disease specialist at King Edward VIII Hospital, recalled, "We never saw gay white men." For Clive Evian, an anti-apartheid stalwart who worked as a doctor in remote clinics in the 1980s, the epidemic was a vague event occurring

21

elsewhere. "I was working in a rural area and it wasn't really an issue for us. It was this Western-oriented illness, gay men. I didn't take very much notice of it."

For Evian, as well as others deeply involved in the anti-apartheid struggle, political commitments fostered their inattention to the unfolding events in Cape Town's and Johannesburg's gay populations. For Clarence Mini, a Black South African who had gone abroad and underground in 1976 and who had been sent by the exiled African National Congress to study medicine in Sofia, Bulgaria, AIDS was perceived through a Cold War filter. "It was their disease, not ours. We preferred to think that there was no homosexuality in Africa; it was a Western homosexual disease."

An activist in NAMDA and then in the United Democratic Front, Jerry Coovadia had been a victim of a police bombing of his home in 1989. At the medical school of the University of Natal, he was seen by students as a courageous public opponent of apartheid and a protector of activist students. For him, AIDS among gay men was an insignificant issue at a time when he and his comrades struggled against a regime bent on destroying their liberation movement and as they confronted the medical afflictions of the impoverished Black, Indian, and Colored populations. That political organizations in the gay community, whatever there were of them, focused almost entirely on securing legal rights for gay white men while avoiding any confrontation with the apartheid order could not help but shape Coovadia's perspective.[1]

> I knew vaguely about HIV, but just vaguely. I know more about SARS
> [severe acute respiratory syndrome] now than I did about HIV then,
> because it wasn't my problem. Why should I be bothered about white
> gay males whose disease was related to their homosexuality? It seemed so
> distant from my own interest. And we had so many big battles to fight,
> that I had absolutely no interest in it, none whatsoever. It just seemed to
> be a problem of gay men. I had never met gay men in my life.

The Epidemic Unfolds

The first reported cases of AIDS in South Africa were diagnosed in 1982. Two men in their early 40s, stewards on South African Air's international flights, had almost certainly been infected through sexual contact with gay men in the United States.[2] Both had experienced a cascade of severe illnesses and died shortly after their admission to intensive care units in Pretoria. They were harbingers of an epidemic that would spread among gay men in Cape Town, Johannesburg, and, to a lesser extent, elsewhere in South Africa. Although the official count rose slowly, by 1985 a pioneering AIDS clinician in Cape Town, Frank Spracklen, and his colleagues would report in the *South African Medical Journal*, the official publication of the

South African Medical Association, "[HIV] infection presents a growing and serious threat to public health.... It has produced a rapidly mounting epidemic among homosexual men, primarily because of their promiscuity, propensity to infection and travel to countries such as the USA."[3]

Observers in South Africa quickly labeled the disease an import. Two years after the initial cases were reported, leading AIDS researchers wrote in the *South African Medical Journal*, "Our data ... suggest that the agent implicated in the causation of AIDS ... is not endemic in southern Africa."[4] Gay men, too, perceived AIDS as an alien threat, provoking feelings of alarm and even hostility toward "outsiders" and those who had sex with them. David Johnson, another early AIDS doctor and, like Miller, a gay man, recalled, "There was a lot of antagonism. The mentality of people was 'these guys mustn't bring it back here; we are so clean.'" He also remembered the suspicion with which a lover of his had been regarded. When Johnson was in his 20s, he had been involved with

a guy who had spent many years in Russia and later America. I remember when that was over, one of my friends came to me and said that another of our friends was having sex with this guy. He said maybe I should tell this guy not to do anything with our friend, because he didn't want this foreigner to bring AIDS to our community. So there was tremendous anger.

Gay Repression in Apartheid South Africa

Like gay men in more liberal societies, those in South Africa were socially and legally vulnerable. But the repressiveness of the apartheid regime gave a special character to the homophobia they were forced to endure. The dominant Afrikaner culture was deeply conservative and religious. Homosexuality was viewed as sinful and as threatening to the moral fiber of the society the National Party sought to build. Under the common law in South Africa, homosexual activity between men was illicit, always subject to harassment by the police.

Following a raid on a private party in Johannesburg and the arrest of guests in drag, the South African Parliament passed new legislation in 1969 that subjected to criminal sanction "any male person who commits with another male person at a party any act which is calculated to stimulate sexual passion or give sexual gratification."[5] In what would become an object of derision among gay men, the act defined a "party" as "any occasion where more than two persons are present."[6] In the wake of that legislation, gays adopted protective maneuvers to avoid arrest. Dennis Sifris, a gay doctor and early AIDS treater in Johannesburg and, like Miller and Johnson, a private practitioner today, recalled that era, a time when he was still in his 20s.

There were one or two clubs opening up in the late 60s where gay
people could go, but there were warning lights. The police raided often,
and suddenly the lights would go on, bright lights, and everybody would
grab the nearest girl! We met, and it was all very private and discreet.

Such homophobia was not restricted to white conservative South Africans,
whether English or Afrikaner. Edwin Cameron, currently a prominent jurist in
South Africa who was named by President Mandela to the High Court in 1994 at
age 41, was, in the 1980s, a leading human rights lawyer. A gay man, he noted the
hostility to gay people within the liberation movement itself. "In 1987, the ANC
representative in London made some quite strident homophobic comments, saying
that gays don't need equal rights. They have all got swimming pools; it's only white
people."[7] It was the outraged response of the ANC's supporters in Europe that
forced its leadership to distance itself officially from such attitudes.

The remark of ANC's London representative echoed statements made by some
Black nationalists that homosexuality was absent in traditional African communities. It was a contamination associated with a colonial system of male labor exploitation, an expression of Western decadence.[8]

That many physicians would share the conservative sexual values of the
broader society is not surprising. What is striking, however, was their willingness
to give public voice to their homophobic views. In a letter to the *South African
Medical Journal* provoked by a clinical report on HIV transmission it had published, a professor at Cape Town's leading hospital, Groote Schuur, wrote, "Surely
the link between dissemination of AIDS and the perverted practices of promiscuous homosexuals is common knowledge.... Who is to know how this self-
confessed pervert achieved his HIV infestation, and are the sordid details really
relevant?"[9] A decade later, when concerns about an extensive heterosexual epidemic
had begun to mount, the head of infectious disease at Johannesburg Hospital
would express similar views. "Once a person denies the authority of the laws of
almighty God, ... he can easily violate all the laws of morality. He can descend into
the amoral abyss, as contemporary events demonstrate." To confront AIDS, it was
necessary to establish "a prohibition of sexual immorality, including adultery,
incest, homosexuality and bestiality."[10]

Less virulent were the comments of a psychiatrist consulted by Steven Miller,
who, at one point in his medical studies, suffered from depression. When asked
about his long-term ambitions, Miller replied that he wanted to become a surgeon,
to which his psychiatrist responded, "Well you can't be homosexual, because
surgery is such a masculine job." Even the admired AIDS pioneer Ruben Sher, who
as an older physician did much to confront public fears and homophobia as he
began his investigations into the new disease with Miller and Sifris, said of gay
men at one point that he did not "agree with their practices." Within that context of pervasive homophobia, the three gay men who would serve as the core of
Johannesburg's medical response to AIDS took individual routes to coming out.

Born in 1945, Dennis Sifris, the oldest of the trio, had chosen, in the 1960s, to keep his desires hidden from his family by maintaining a heterosexual façade.

> They didn't know. They didn't know. I had the odd girlfriend now and then. Luckily I met a young Jewish girl who was a lesbian. It was perfect for me; for four or five years we went out. She was my girlfriend, and I met her parents. We went out and used to go to gay places and the gay clubs, and she attracted all the boys, which was wonderful!

Within his family, Sifris's homosexuality was never spoken of. "I never actually told my mother," Sifris confessed, "but she knew." After she died, he recalled, his father drove him to the airport and expressed his longing for grandchildren:

> "Well, now your mother's dead, it was her dying wish that you get married and have children and settle down." And I turned to him and I said, "Listen Dad, there's no such nonsense as dying wishes. And I will get married, but not to a woman; it will be to a man." To which his father replied, "So what time are you coming back?"

Miller told a very different story. Almost ten years younger than Sifris, he was open with his parents and those who were important to him, as he struggled with the "marginalizing experience of being gay." However, only with a trip to the United States in 1976 as part of his medical training was he able to appreciate fully how socially oppressive South Africa was:

> It was my first trip outside the country and in retrospect it was extremely important because that was the era of gay liberation in the U.S. And while I can't say I was more than a gay interested onlooker, the rightness of it and just the common sense of it really got to me. I came back to South Africa filled with the desire to make things change.

Looking back on how he acted subsequently, he was struck by how brash and perhaps "silly" he became:

> They were kind of in-your-face stuff. I had a button on my white coat that said "How dare you assume I'm heterosexual." And I wore makeup to medical school, which was probably not a good idea. I tried to set up an organization at the university along the lines of the then-fledgling American gay student groups, and it was just seen as someone's crazy idea.

Miller was fortunate not to be taken seriously. Only a few years earlier, in 1972, an effort on the part of gay students at the University of Natal in Durban to create a campus organization, the South African Gay Liberation Movement, was quickly squelched by the police. Since sodomy was a common-law offense, the movement would be breaking the law, according to the authorities, by inciting people to illicit activity.[11]

For David Johnson, the youngest of the three gay doctors, coming out in the 1980s was still something that had to be approached with care. "There was a lot of gay bashing, a lot of discrimination. One was always wary of who one would come out to."

First Response: Facing Resistance and Denial

It was against this backdrop that the gay response to the new epidemic took shape. Gay AIDS activists faced formidable barriers as they made initial efforts to provide community support for care and prevention. Because homosexuality was still illegal, it was even difficult to raise money. "One needed to get a fundraising number," Steven Miller remembered:

> And the government quite openly said we do not give fundraising numbers to criminals. So the only way around that was that, from time to time, other registered organizations, particularly a group called the Witwatersrand Mental Health Society in Johannesburg, would permit some group to piggyback on their fundraising number and raise a little bit of cash.

As frustrating was the denial that persisted among gay men. The official publication of the Gay Association of South Africa, *Link/Skakel*, headlined in early 1983, "AIDS Panic Is Overstressed."[12] In an article that was not too different from many that had appeared in other countries at the start of the AIDS epidemic, the newspaper went on to report the views of the executive chairman of the gay association: "While the seriousness ... cannot be denied, AIDS hasn't by any stretch of the imagination reached epidemic proportions."[13]

In the 1980s, when homosexuality had to remain secretive, largely hidden indoors, gay meeting places were especially important. When Dennis Sifris attempted to raise awareness about AIDS, he sought out such gay establishments:

> In '83, we decided we were going to go to the popular gay club, the Venue, on a Saturday night. We asked them permission to put a little table outside with our safe sex and awareness pamphlets. We had condoms and the usual sort of thing you see in every gay bar in the States. And nobody even came; they sort of looked and pulled away—that was the reaction. At 12:30, I went to the owner and said, "I want to say a few words." They stopped the music, turned the lights up, and I stood in the middle of the dance floor in a gay club, and I said, "People, you must just listen to me. We've got a problem and this is the AIDS story," and slowly the dance

floor emptied and they all moved away from me. So I just said, "It's a big problem, and we think it's only happening in America but it's happening here, and you've got to be aware. We've got a little stall outside, and we want volunteers, we want people to come up and see if they can volunteer their time to help us." No response. I think three people came. I still feel that feeling of standing in the middle of a disco, speaking, telling them it's not a police raid, it's actually more of an emergency.

In the first years of the epidemic, as Sifris sought to educate the gay community, creating the AIDS Action Group for that purpose, Ruben Sher, who was a physician-investigator at the South African Institute for Medical Research (SAIMR) in Johannesburg, discovered a new direction for his scientific work. Sher had completed a Ph.D. in immunology in 1980. A visit to the United States in 1982 to seek medical care for his son brought him into contact with the then-emerging challenge of AIDS. News accounts in the American press, as well as meetings with researchers at the National Institutes of Health and at the Centers for Disease Control, sparked his interest in the new disease. At a time when no one understood what was causing the recently named acquired immune deficiency syndrome, the prospect of investigating the immunological status of gay men seemed both critically important and exciting.

After his return to South Africa, Sher spoke with Steven Miller, who was working at SAIMR, a center for infectious disease research since 1914,[14] and contacted Dennis Sifris, with whom he had previously conducted prevalence studies on hepatitis B in gay men. It seemed only logical to use Sifris's private practice and wider contacts in his community to recruit research subjects. But Sher went further in broadcasting his interest in studying gay men. Quarraisha Abdool Karim, already a microbiologist but training under Sher at the time, recalled:

> Steven and Ruben put adverts in the newspaper and went on radio, and we would have queues of gay men from all over South Africa and beyond coming through to undergo an examination. We took blood, sexual histories, and we ran every serological assay that we had in the lab. It was really a fishing expedition. These men were coming in healthy, and all we were trying to do was to construct who they were and expose their body fluids to whatever laboratory tests were available.

In taking this step, Sher was laying the groundwork for ongoing surveillance of both AIDS and occult infection with HIV. Once he gained access to the first viral antibody test in 1985, he assayed the stored sera of the 250 gay men examined in 1983 and found that almost 13 percent were already infected.[15] At the same time, he created the first clinical setting in Johannesburg for counseling men at risk, a precursor of the system of voluntary testing and counseling that would in time emerge at many sites in South Africa.

Because everyone was faced with sheer uncertainty, the relationships between those who came to the clinic and its professional staff underwent a radical shift; doctors unable to cure had no alternative but to care. Of that time, Abdool Karim recalled:

> This was the first time where the doctor-patient relationship was actually
> altered because the doctors who were trying to help were as much in
> the dark [as the patients]. We had people who were very worried. What
> they needed was counseling and support; so they would come there,
> and what they wanted to do was talk.

This experience would shape her ideas about what counseling and testing should be like when, a decade later, as a government official, she had to address AIDS in the immediate period following the election of Nelson Mandela as president. "What people needed was just a sympathetic ear."

What left a lasting impression on her was not just the fact that the clinic was engaged in pioneering work. She was struck additionally by the spirit of Sher's clinic. "The thing that I learned from working there was about humanity and humaneness. While everybody was running away in fear, Ruben and Steven were saying, 'Well, we don't know what's going on, but let's look at it.'" Although Abdool Karim was not a doctor, Sher taught her something important about what it meant to be a clinician. "You [didn't] know whether you were going to get exposed or not, and here was Ruben saying, 'Come one, come all.'" Sher himself said of that period, "To me, they were patients. Their background didn't make any difference. They were people dying of a very interesting disease."

Not only was the clinic open to gay people, whether patients or staff, it was also unlike the racially divided world of work in South Africa. As an Indian woman who had grown up under apartheid, Abdool Karim knew that in the 1980s:

> Many of the workplaces had separate toilets for Black and white workers.
> The tea rooms were also separated. But at the institute we were fairly
> integrated. For the first time, I felt I was living in a nonracial envi-
> ronment, and so it was the humanity that kept us together.

Sher's efforts took place within the relatively liberal academic-medical atmosphere of the University of Witwatersrand in Johannesburg. In fact, Abdool Karim recalled that despite the pervasive stigma that surrounded both homosexuality and the new disease, the dean of the medical school led a public memorial service for a young gay doctor who died of AIDS in the late 1980s. But such gestures could go only so far.

In a country where denial and discrimination were so common, it became difficult, even for prominent and professionally successful individuals, to come to terms with a diagnosis of AIDS. Working at Baragwanath Hospital in Soweto,

Glenda Gray recalled how her supervisor and mentor, a gay man, had fought the demons raised by HIV: degenerative illness, stigma, fear of disclosure, and death.

> He vacillated from being in complete denial to looking at alternative
> medicine; he started running to improve his health and took homeopathic
> remedies. He struggled because he was from a Catholic family, and even
> at his funeral, no one mentioned that he had died of AIDS.

Gray's account of her mentor's personal desperation was echoed by Edwin Cameron, who learned in 1986, when he was working as a public interest and human rights lawyer at the University of Witwatersrand, that he was infected with HIV. Late on a Friday afternoon, he received a call from his physician, who informed him of his diagnosis. The shock was all the greater since he had never been told that his blood was being tested for the virus.

> It was undoubtedly the worst shock I have ever received in my life, and
> it was classically bad practice. It was on the telephone, he was 60 kilometers
> away in Pretoria, and it was a Friday afternoon at 4 o'clock. All he said
> to me was that there is someone at the Institute of Medical Research,
> Dr. Ruben Sher, who you may want to consult with at some time. So he
> left me resourceless. It was the most frightful experience, and it has
> given me a very personal sense of what a violation unconsented testing
> involved, especially uncounseled testing, and the effect on me was
> very profound.

Cameron kept the news to himself, turning to neither friends nor family. Most amazing to him, as he recalled that moment in his life, was that it took him three years to disclose his diagnosis to his sister, with whom he was very close.

> I felt filthy, I felt guilty, I felt contaminated, and I felt unable to deal
> with the horror of the infection. I also felt unable to burden my family with
> it; at the same time, I felt unable to deal with the burden of their responses.
> It was a terrible pity, because when eventually I did speak to them, I
> received unhesitatingly loving responses. And I still think that if the test had
> been planned and counseled, I might have been able to speak to them
> earlier.

Too ashamed to talk about his condition, too fearful of the responses of colleagues and clients, it took Cameron more than a decade to make the political and ethical decision to announce publicly that he was infected. His action, he believed, made him among the first high officials in Africa to reveal their HIV status.

Ironically, Cameron's introduction to advocacy on behalf of those who were HIV infected was a consequence neither of his status as a gay man nor as a patient but in his professional capacity as a human rights lawyer. In his memoir, *Witness to AIDS*, he recounted:

> In August 1986, the mine bosses' organization, the Chamber of Mines,
> announced the results of a study of blood samples of 300,000 male
> mineworkers. These showed about 800 mineworkers—760 of whom were
> from central Africa, in particular Malawi—had HIV. The reaction was
> drastic. The workers with HIV were summarily deported. . . . Regardless
> of their years of service, they were sent back to Malawi—with its pitifully
> inadequate health system—to meet their fate. It was this issue, brought
> to me because I was a human rights lawyer doing trade union work, that
> drew me into AIDS policy and litigation.[16]

The shame experienced by Cameron and by Glenda Gray's mentor was buttressed by the official posture of the South African government, which was beginning to respond to the AIDS epidemic in the mid-1980s. Because he was a physician treating public and private patients with a new disease, and because of his special insights as a gay man, Dennis Sifris believed that he would have much to contribute to the AIDS Advisory Group, created in 1985, which provided expert medical advice to the minister of health. The group was chaired by the director of the South African Institute for Medical Research and included Ruben Sher. When Sifris requested membership, he was unceremoniously turned down.

> I applied for the AIDS Advisory Group, and they said, "No, we can't
> have you, because you represent one of the high-risk groups, and if we have
> a homosexual, you've got to have a prostitute, and, God forbid, a Black
> person." So I wasn't on the AIDS Advisory Group. And I was not happy
> with that.

Steven Miller also recalled the frustration of being excluded from that advisory body, which dealt with issues so intimately important to him.

> The members of the AIDS Advisory Group, I honestly cannot remember
> them all, were representatives from the blood bank, obviously policy
> makers from the Health Department, virologists, and Ruben Sher. In fact, in
> the entire history of the AIDS Advisory Group, there was never repre-
> sentation from any of the affected groups. This was a cabal of grey-suited
> men, who told the minister all that she wanted to hear. Essentially, the
> official line on HIV became, as the minister of health then publicly
> said, "HIV and AIDS are indicative of poor social behavior."

Not surprisingly, the government refused to provide any financial support to fledging gay community groups. Ironically, the unmet needs of the Black impoverished population would be used to justify rejecting the gay men's appeals for support. When Dennis Sifris, leading a group of gay men, approached the Department of Health about obtaining resources for AIDS prevention efforts, he was told by its director: "It's very interesting, gentlemen, but AIDS is not a problem in this country, TB is a problem. I'm sorry; we haven't got money to help you." Such views were augmented by the AIDS Advisory Group, which, concerned about preventing unreasonable fear of contagion, sought to minimize the importance of AIDS. "We must view AIDS realistically," the group's director asserted in 1985. The number of reported cases was still relatively small compared to other diseases. "[Since 1983] we had 60,000 reported cases of tuberculosis."[17]

Official denial of the gravity of the emerging epidemic was mirrored by the indifference of Sifris's colleagues. When he brought a veteran of the American AIDS outbreak in San Francisco to the Johannesburg Hospital, the visitor was met with derision by members of the Department of Medicine. Bearded and wearing sandals, appearing before an audience clad in white coats and ties, he could easily be set apart, his message quickly denigrated. "They all sort of laughed, and they thought, well, it's a disease among queers in San Francisco. It's not our problem."

Restricting Care

Johannesburg Hospital itself sought to close its doors to those who were suffering from AIDS. Describing what would become all too common in South Africa's response to this disease, Miller underscored how limited resources could provide the rationalization for the denial of care.

> It was very difficult to get people admitted. There was a great reluctance because it was seen as someone with an inevitably fatal condition, and there were other things competing. And it was a teaching hospital where HIV was not seen as having value for instructional purposes. It was really wasting everybody's time.

When the sick did gain access to the wards, it was commonly through the emergency room. And then, a refusal to confront the gravity of what was unfolding could take the form of stark denial and neglect. Miller recalled when a senior colleague refused to acknowledge what laboratory results had made clear.

> I remember the first time when we saw *Pneumocystis carinii* pneumonia [PCP]. I did the stain and looked at it, and this was *Pneumocystis.* But the professor of respiratory medicine said, "*Pneumocystis* doesn't happen in Africa. So it's not *Pneumocystis.*" But it was; it was right there.

On the wards, concerns about resource limitations would provide the rationale for imposing strictures on the use of services. Although he would go on to become a doctor working in rural KwaZulu-Natal, Bernhard Gaede was a 22-year-old nurse-in-training at Johannesburg Hospital during the early years of the AIDS epidemic. What he experienced as cruel unwillingness to address the needs of a gay man with AIDS left a lasting memory:

> I remember there was a quiet hush amongst the nursing staff. This was
> an AIDS patient. You couldn't talk loud about it; you had to whisper when
> you said the word. And I was allocated to nurse him. I really liked him.
> When the ward wasn't very busy, I had quite a lot of time to speak with
> him; he was quite ill. We talked a lot about where he was at, and of his
> sister, who wasn't visiting him, something which caused him a huge
> amount of pain. He had bad diarrhea. We had to change the linen all
> the time, and he was really upset by being so debilitated and dependent on
> people. One time, he was crying and crying, and I was sitting there listening
> to him, and the senior sister walks in and said, "Oh, you're sitting down.
> What do you think you're doing?" I was just so angry. So I said, "I am
> practicing holistic patient care." And she said, "You're getting smart," and
> waltzed off.

Opposing limits on service to men with AIDS did not simply pit doctors and nurses committed to their care against those antagonistic to meeting their needs. Rather, advocates for extending care to gay men who had fallen ill had to confront a consensus that in public hospitals it was crucial to husband already scarce resources. Ian Sanne, whose holistic medical world view was shaped by Rudolph Steiner's philosophy of theosophy, recalled that as an intern in the early 1990s he learned about both the disease and the need to justify using scarce resources.

> In my intern year, I started coming into contact more readily with pa-
> tients who were HIV positive and, in fact, had an aversion—a fear—of
> treating HIV patients. They tended to be gay white males who were at the
> end of their lives, presenting with florid infections or leukemia or lympho-
> mas that were fairly untreatable. It always really felt like a complete disaster
> and not really salvageable. At the same time, within that hopelessness, I
> definitely had an attitude of assisting people with pain and suffering. It
> was never a question that they lie in the corner of the ward and I wouldn't
> do anything about it.
>   And then I had a very formative experience. A young man came to
> the ward, and it turned out that he and I had actually been friends
> in nursery school, and since nursery school we hadn't known each other.
> He presented with PCP pneumonia. His consciousness was completely

normal, but he was incredibly breathless. We decided to ventilate him. This turned into a ventilation procedure of about 14 days with major infection control problems within the ward. The nursing staff was up in arms about this. The continuous fight to actually keep this person on the ward and ventilated led to a viewpoint where I basically felt that these very late-stage patients in our environment with limited resources should not be accessing intensive care.

Fear of contagion, often based on ignorance of how HIV was transmitted, contributed to the kind of treatment experienced by AIDS patients. Repeating patterns that occurred worldwide in the early years of this epidemic, extraordinary measures were taken to erect barriers between the sick and those who would be called to care for them. These demoralizing practices persisted in South Africa, even as evidence began to emerge about what protective measures were, in fact, necessary. As in the United States, doctors who used invasive procedures, surgeons in particular, were especially wary of treating HIV-infected individuals. Frank Spracklen, speaking in 1988 at the first major meeting on AIDS held in Johannesburg, reported that only one doctor in Cape Town was willing to do bronchoscopies on infected patients; and only one pathologist was willing to do postmortems on those who had died of AIDS. Dennis Sifris added that the head of infectious disease at a major hospital in the then-Transvaal refused to have anything to do with HIV patients.[18] Such attitudes would persist. A study in Cape Town in the early 1990s found that more than 70 percent of anesthetists believed that they had a right to refuse to treat patients with HIV infection.[19]

The pages of the *South African Medical Journal* were filled at the time—and later—with letters justifying such refusals. Lamenting the fate of physicians in the public sector, one doctor wrote, "A private practitioner is entitled to choose his patients to a certain extent, . . . but the state-employed doctor has no such right. Does the idea of informed consent not apply to medical personnel, or are they obliged to undertake any risk because they are state owned?"[20]

At Baragwanath Hospital, the head of surgery, Professor Bernard (Bokkie) Rabinowitz,[21] put up a sign which read: "If you are to undergo an operation, you must understand that you're going to have an [HIV] test." He would not operate on those who were infected. Rabinowitz's actions were the subject of controversy among the faculty and students at the medical school. Dennis Sifris described those times:

There was nothing we could do about it. I remember one debate at the medical school with Bokkie Rabinowitz on one side, who is a very dynamic surgeon, and the head of ethics. And Bokkie won hands down. All the medical students voted for him, because he presented their viewpoint, putting ourselves at risk, putting our wives at risk, putting our children at risk, etc.

As Sifris, aware of the international scientific consensus about what was needed to protect caregivers from their patients' infections, approached his sick patients on the wards of Johannesburg Hospital, the main teaching hospital serving the Witwatersrand medical school, he was outraged by the shields that had been erected.

> They were sick boys. And I remember, when I went to visit them, there were the double gloves, the double gowns, and the big spaceman thing, and I would go in without anything on. I would say, "Take this away, take this away." I pulled down all the barriers and pulled them away, and told the mothers and fathers to take off the gloves and touch the patient.

The nurses often resisted his demands. "I remember having big fights with all the sisters in the wards, because I would come in and say, 'You can't do this.'"

Even at Somerset Hospital in Cape Town, where Frank Spracklen had taken on the care of AIDS patients, pervasive fear characterized the responses of nurses and doctors. Despite his commitment to those with HIV-related conditions, Spracklen himself was not immune to those fears. Felicity Cope, an infectious disease nurse who had come to Cape Town from Zimbabwe in 1970 when she was 26 years old, would assume much of the burden of AIDS education in the institution. She said of Spracklen, "He was frightened of his patients and often used to stand at the door" as he conducted his consultation. She also described what she recalled as the hysterical response of a senior colleague as the first AIDS patients entered Somerset. "She was at her wit's end. She said she couldn't get nurses to go into the wards and she was also very reluctant."

Beyond the everyday burdens created by such refusals, Cope remembered the general atmosphere of fear and disdain toward AIDS that pervaded medicine in Cape Town. She recalled her first encounter with an HIV patient, before she had moved to Somerset Hospital, so searing that its details remained fresh to her two decades later:

> I was about to go home when I got a phone call from the head of the Trauma Unit asking me to clean the unit as a young man who had attempted suicide, one of Dr. Spracklen's patients, had been admitted. The unit head was very agitated because, at that time, Dr. Spracklen was the only physician seeing patients with HIV.

When she arrived in the unit, she found a patient whose

> bones were sticking out all over the place and who was bleeding profusely. They'd resuscitated him and then discovered that he was a Spracklen patient. They wanted to send him to have an x-ray, and none of the porters would take him.

Despite her own fears, Cope took on the challenge she believed her professional responsibilities demanded of her.

> So I put on a gown, and found one person who would help me. Blood was dripping off the trolley. I can remember walking along the corridor, pulling down my gown and thinking, I wonder when I last shaved my legs? I wonder how much blood will go through the stockings? The person who was doing the x-rays was very hassled about it, but he was really good. I had to do all the moving and lifting. I had about three or four pairs of gloves on and my gown, which was material, so how much good was it doing? Then we went to the operating theater, and that's where I met an absolute wall, a brick wall. They wouldn't let me push him into the theater. The anesthetist wouldn't see him and resisted allowing him into the theater. Eventually it went to a higher power, and they had to operate. But the anesthetist just opted out and wouldn't go near him. Dressed in space suits, welding masks, gowns, and waterproofs, they amputated his legs. When he got to the ward, the nurses wouldn't change the dressings. No one wanted to give him a bedpan. No one wanted to do anything for him, so initially I did a lot of the nursing.

Against this backdrop of rejection and stigmatization, a few physicians began to recognize the need to create outpatient clinics that could meet the needs of patients suffering from the new disease. At Johannesburg Hospital, Dennis Sifris approached one of his mentors about these needs. Although he quickly agreed to provide space for such a clinic, it was in a remote, even secluded, location. As Sifris described it, "Level 4, basement 3, third corridor, 'round the corner." Initially the clinic, which was staffed by unpaid volunteers, met only once a month; as demand rose, clinic days increased to once, then twice, a week.

In a move that was not dissimilar to what had occurred in other countries and would recur many times in South Africa, there was an initial effort to protect those attending the clinic by giving it a name designed to mask its purposes. And so the Johannesburg facility was first known as the Immune Disorders Clinic. But Dennis Sifris, its first formal director, was unhappy with such secrecy. "The only way we're going to deal with this is to get open with it, and the doctors have to accept it, and you can't do it all in secret." In 1985, he renamed the service the HIV Clinic. His action produced an uproar. "You're not going to get them coming. They don't want to be known as HIV. We must keep it secret." Sifris remained unswayed.

The experience of those who worked in and depended on the clinic was shaped by the fact that it served gay white men. When hemophiliacs and others who had acquired HIV infection through blood products began to develop AIDS, the hospital provided a separate service for treatment. Steven Miller sardonically recalled that "any attempt that we made to amalgamate the services was absolutely rejected, and the general perception was that it would not be a good idea for hemophiliacs to mix with people who had given them this problem."

For the gay doctors working in Johannesburg, the evolving AIDS epidemic had impacts that were not only professional, but personal as well. As in the United States, these physicians touched their infected patients because others would not. In looking back on that period, Miller mockingly upbraided himself: "Those were the days when you would hug your patients, when there was a great show of physical affection; and that was just very inappropriate. Now someone who comes in with angina, you don't start hugging them." At times, this desire to be better, more caring than other doctors could lead to unforeseen consequences. He recounted an occasion when a dermatologist, called in to examine a patient's rash, observed the condition without touching it. Offended by his insensitivity, the clinic staff reached out to make physical contact with the patient.

> Of course, we were wrong in that situation, because a week later I got scabies and everybody else in the clinic got scabies, a very common condition we see in this country. All of us who were making such an effort to be physically demonstrative got the infection from the patient, and the doctor whom we maligned for putting his hand[s] behind his back and not touching the rash was spared that indignity.

The Limits of Medicine

Miller was acutely aware of the limits of medical treatment.

> We used to try vitamins and herbal supplements and plant extracts and antabuse—used to treat alcoholism—and all of those early putative remedies, none of which in the end proved effective. So you became a person who had to be a good counselor. You had to learn to help people find meaning in the life that they had, none of which we had been trained to do.

He summed up the situation by saying, "It was a wilderness. There were no teachings on the topic of treating AIDS. Nobody knew what was going on, and we would read avidly. We all spent a lot of our own money trying to visit people overseas to learn from them."

Learning was all the more difficult because of the international academic boycott and isolation of South Africa during the last decade of the apartheid regime. The restrictions placed by some countries on granting visas to South Africans made it more difficult for physicians to attend meetings overseas. AIDS experts from abroad who were willing to assist those facing the epidemic in South Africa were so few that their efforts were deemed to be remarkable.

In a country where only a small number of clinicians took on the responsibility of caring for AIDS patients, efforts to advance the understanding of how HIV affected the body's organs could lead to research that was at once too personal and too macabre. Felicity Cope, who so often assumed responsibility for tasks that few others would take on, volunteered to assist a pathologist, Gideon Knobel, as he conducted autopsies to study the brains of those who had died of AIDS. She tearfully recalled:

> I still get fairly hassled about it, because I had got to know these guys and many of them were friends. To extract the brain, he cut the skin across the top of the head from ear to ear and peeled it away from the scalp and forehead, which caused the face to crumple and distort. It was very distressing—the face is so much of the person, it was watching them being mutilated. The face was the person I knew, that was him. We had to be very careful with the knives. He'd cut the cadaver from sternum to pubis and then open it out, and to keep the knife from falling, he would stab it into the leg. It was the safest thing to do, and after all the leg is not feeling it. I couldn't eat or cook or have anything to do with meat; I would become a vegetarian for a few days after each one. Often, I'd go home and cry my eyes out.

Unlike Knobel, whom she described as having only a scant acquaintance with the patients in the autopsy room, Cope brought with her the personal ties she had developed and treasured. Like the gay doctors who bore the burden of caring for AIDS patients in the 1980s, crossing professional boundaries that would normally provide emotional distance was not uncommon for her.

> If you wanted, you could have nothing to do with the patients. You could say, that patient has an infection, and forget the face, forget they were people. But that's defeating the object. Also you become friendly with the patients. A lot of them became really good friends. A lot of them I mixed with socially as well.

Because nothing could be done about the underlying infection, Cope's patients were repeatedly admitted to the wards. It was such ongoing, although intermittent, contact that served to intensify her relationships. These had a bittersweet quality, because death was inevitable.

> I got to a stage where I said, "I'll have to actually get out of this, because everybody I work with dies." All my patients die. I've got this whole group of people, and you learn to like them, you get to know them, you get to know their good and their bad and everything, and you know they're going to die.

By the late 1980s, Dennis Sifris and Steven Miller in Johannesburg had seen between them almost 600 patients, at least 60 percent of whom had already died. Looming for them was the fear of how much worse things could get, since they believed that as many as 15,000 gay men in the Johannesburg region alone had HIV infection.[22] In recalling those years, Miller spoke of how emotionally depleting the situation had been.

> Part of dealing with people with HIV was, I suppose, being paternal, trying
> to be the almost perpetually protecting parent for a lot of people. We
> became involved in all aspects of the patients' lives, their relationships,
> their homes, their financial situations. We would go out at night. We would
> sit with people, we would do house calls, we would be there when the
> person took his or her last breath.

The bonds that Sifris and Miller formed with their patients drew on a sense of shared danger for their community and themselves. "It was extraordinarily difficult because all of us, myself included," said Miller,

> became overinvolved with every single patient. To an extent, I suspect,
> there was a lot of personal identification. There was a sense of, there but for
> the grace of God go all of us; and there was this real sense of unfairness.
> It really just was bad luck that someone had got it or good luck that a
> person had avoided the infection.

Ironically, the fact that he himself was free of HIV was an additional burden.

> I had a very bizarre sense of grief at not being infected or the sense
> of feeling different; somehow I wasn't good enough. I wasn't authentic
> in some way, because here was I, the HIV negative person, working
> in a world of people with an illness that affected us all so profoundly.
> Yet I was the one who was going home and knowing, well, I didn't
> have it; so I think there was a huge amount of guilt at being HIV
> negative.

The omnipresence of death made Miller and his colleagues feel especially vulnerable, both personally and professionally. There was so little they could do as doctors, and yet it was difficult for them to admit defeat. "You had someone who was bright and vibrant and full of life, and certain parts of you were saying, but this is someone who is dead, but not just yet." For Miller, living in the face of such anticipation created "an overwhelming need to make it better and OK for that person, even if it consumed all of you." Such devotion and the eventual losses took their toll, he recalled.

It was just a profound depth of despair and depression with nobody to provide support for the caregivers. So it was an extremely difficult time. We would try and talk with colleagues about it, but doctors weren't really interested in issues of death and dying. Each death made one more vulnerable; and at the same time it gave one more resolve to fight this. But part of oneself became much, much more vulnerable, and it became difficult working with HIV for that reason. I think we all went through periods where we just felt we could not face another sick person, but we had to, and we just had to push on because if the two or three or four of us who were doing the work weren't around, perhaps in an omnipotent way, we felt, well, the situation was going to become disastrous. I think it reflected how intensely we became embroiled in this, perhaps to an unhealthy degree, and how few other resources there were. At times, I wouldn't even use other services that were available, hospice, for example. In a sense, we saw hospice as a failure of our own individual ability to give the patient a good death.

As in the United States, the desire of AIDS doctors to provide the "good death," one with dignity and without pain, led some to help their patients and friends to commit suicide. One doctor who was particularly committed to assisting those with AIDS when they could no longer tolerate their suffering had come to an agreement with a friend that he would help him end his life when the time came. Late one night, when death appeared imminent, he was called.

When I arrived, my friend couldn't move in the bed. All he did was give a weak smile. He couldn't really talk, just said, "Thank you." I and my boyfriend sat with him for a few minutes, chatting. Then the patient's parents arrived. I said I had to give him something for pain. I took a needle, a morphine amp, and said, "I'm putting some in here for him." I put up the drip and openly wept. Within minutes, the patient's mother said she thought he had stopped breathing. Of course, everyone fell apart then. It had been hard to do, particularly because the patient was a friend. The patient's mother, who was a simple woman, who everyone described as terribly discriminatory, came to where I and my boyfriend were hugging each other and sobbing. She put her hand on my leg and said, "Such a shame; I understand how you feel. You're just two queers like him." She was incredible. She said, "Don't worry; you're OK."

At times, death could cut even closer. For Dennis Sifris, who was himself infected with HIV, the death of his lover remained a powerful memory.

He was Swedish, and he was being looked after in Sweden, and went back and forth twice a year. He had a few Kaposi's lesions on his foot. And he was not too well; we were going back to Sweden to see his doctors and to see his family. We were sitting at the Brussels airport in the transit lounge, and he suddenly said, "Oh, I have such pain in my head." So I said, "Let's go on the plane. It's noisy here." And he couldn't get up. We had a wheelchair, and by the time we got on the plane, I said, "You must get up and walk to seat number one." He couldn't, and he died, on the plane. He died in Brussels, and I took him home to his family. That was ten years ago. I've lived with it.

Transitions

When the first antiviral drug, AZT (Zidovudine), was licensed in 1986, it marked an important milestone in the clinical response to AIDS in North America and Europe. But when it was first marketed, AZT was extraordinarily expensive, even in the United States, where it cost approximately $10,000 a year. When it arrived in South Africa in 1987, only the most privileged could afford what was thought to be a life-saving medication. For Steven Miller, it was both a turning point and a moral problem.

> I remember the day very well when we got AZT. I was sitting in a clinic and the representative from its manufacturer, Burroughs-Wellcome, came in with this bottle with little white capsules with a little blue ring around it. We all held these in our hands and thought, the miracle is here. None of our patients could afford the original price for the recommended 1200 milligrams a day. Since there was no science in antiretroviral therapy, we decided we would halve the dose. I remember speaking to an expert in England about this, and he acted as though we were crazy.

As head of the HIV clinic at Johannesburg Hospital from 1985 until 1990, Dennis Sifris also anguished over the price of the new drug. He noted:

> We were at least able to offer AZT to our patients who could afford it, because there was a big social mix. Then the hospital decided that the hemophiliacs who were innocent victims of this epidemic would get AZT. So I reacted to that. Why are the hemophiliacs getting AZT free when my patients are not?

Outraged, Sifris gave an interview which made clear his dismay at the discriminatory hospital policies. "Within a day or two, I was summoned to the hospital superintendent's office, who said, 'We have to go meet the secretary of health in Pretoria.' I was reprimanded severely because as an employee of the hospital, I had no right to criticize its policies." Shortly thereafter, Sifris resigned.

His place was taken by Miller, who faced a similar battle. A patient in his clinic who was going blind because of an opportunistic disorder, CMV (cytomegalovirus) retinitis, was denied access to ganciclovir, the one drug that could reverse his condition. At the same time, the hospital was offering this medication to cancer patients. He backed his patient, who had successfully brought his case to court. "The reason I left the clinic was that I was told to go, because I had supported a patient's legal claim. I became persona non grata. I had no official post; I wasn't being paid. It was time to go, and the door was closed."

His successor, David Spencer, a seasoned infectious disease specialist just returned from a fellowship at the Cleveland Clinic in the United States, was sent into the clinic by hospital officials as a way of regaining control from gay doctors. He had no more luck as an advocate. Ultimately, he too resigned in protest. Spencer described sitting at meetings with the hospital's chief pharmacist, requesting medication for those with CMV retinitis. After what he felt were interminable discussions, he would be told that it was a decision to be made in Pretoria by the national government, "and that went on until these guys were totally blind or died. And it was like a game. One reason I eventually left was that you were castrated by the whole process; you had no way of getting anywhere."

Each of the doctors who had pioneered HIV work ultimately turned away from the public sector, developing large private AIDS practices. Ironically, their departures coincided with the emerging awareness of what would become a vast Black heterosexual epidemic, which would both overwhelm the memory of the country's first encounter with AIDS and impose ever-greater demands on South Africa's state-supported hospitals and clinics.

The first Black South African heterosexual AIDS cases—two women who had never left the rural Transvaal—were diagnosed in late 1987.[23] A study of miners by Ruben Sher at the South African Institute for Medical Research the year before had revealed an HIV infection rate of 3.8 percent in Malawian workers, but no infections among their South African counterparts. In a 1989 review article in the *South African Medical Journal*, he warned about the increase in the Black population of AIDS cases, which had reached 22 in December 1988, including 3 children.[24] By October 1989, the cumulative number of reported Black AIDS cases had risen to 40.[25] At Durban's King Edward VIII Hospital, in one 15-month period, 9 children were diagnosed with HIV infection.[26] While these numbers were small and, in hindsight, only a fraction of the true prevalence, it was clear that the rate of increase presaged the emergence of a potential catastrophe in a Black population that previously had been free of HIV. By the end of 1989, seroprevalence in some parts of the country was already close to 1 percent.[27] The relative protection that had been afforded to South Africa by its political isolation was ending. One analysis concluded that as many as 400,000 Black South Africans would be infected by 1992 and that millions of South Africans might die of AIDS in the coming decades.[28]

In warning of the possibility of a "biological holocaust," Ruben Sher urged readers of the *South African Medical Journal* to ask themselves: "'How many more people must die before we do something about this disease?' A pre-emptive strike is needed now; in 5 years' time it will be too late."[29] His anxiety was echoed by other experts observing the evolving epidemiology of HIV in South Africa. "The HIV/AIDS epidemic constitutes the greatest threat to public health in South Africa this century. The control of the epidemic is a question of national importance, and may quite possibly become a question of national survival."[30] Ironically, just as amnesia would set in regarding the gay AIDS epidemic in South Africa, these dire and alarming predictions would be all but forgotten by those who took up the burden of AIDS treatment in the mid- and late 1990s.

2

Facing AIDS

Denial, Indifference, and Fear

First Signs

The second South African epidemic emerged slowly, like water seeping languidly to the surface. Raziya Bobat, a pediatrician born in Durban in 1954 and trained in its "nonwhite" medical school, encountered her first AIDS patient in 1987 at King Edward VIII Hospital at about the same time as the first Black cases appeared in the Transvaal. Only recently aware that AIDS existed in South Africa, she had just begun reading about the disease, when one of her colleagues alerted her to an anomalous case:

> She was an African child about five years old; 99 percent of our patients are Black African. Our specialist had looked at the skin and said that there was something strange about this child; and the more she looked at her, the more she seemed to fit this description that everybody was talking about, about HIV. Of course, then all of us looked at this kid; then we took out the books and we read about it. And everybody sort of said, "Yeah, this certainly seems like it."

It was also in 1987 that James McIntyre, then 31 years old and working on the vast campus of Baragwanath Hospital, serving the populous Black township of Soweto, had to grapple with a deeply disturbing piece of news. Already aware, as a gay man, of the extent of infection in his own community, he now faced laboratory evidence that HIV was making its presence felt in the impoverished populations he treated.

> The South African Blood Transfusion Service brought in their test kits and decided to try them on some stored blood specimens that they had from us

43

and found, to their shock and horror, that some of them were positive for the HIV antibody. They didn't know what to do because there was no patient consent. There had been no discussion with anybody at that stage. Worried about the women, we then called them back in.

His colleague in pediatrics, Glenda Gray, saw her first HIV case, a Black child, a year later. Slowly she was discovering AIDS, case by case, in her township patients. "We started seeing a few, occasionally," she said. "But, basically, it was quite rare at that stage." Also at Baragwanath in those years was another politically committed doctor, Saul Johnson, who was involved with the ANC underground in the late 1980s and remembered a trickle of HIV cases and a flood of other diseases in Soweto. "I saw very little HIV disease. I think we were starting to see a little bit of pediatric disease, because the pediatric disease clinically pre-dates the adult disease."

It was not easy to identify those first cases. Although AIDS had been treated in South African gay men for over five years, most doctors, given their specialties, the segregation of hospitals by race, and their avoidance of the gay epidemic, had no experience with the disease. Henry Sunpath, who would eventually assume a leadership role in the care of AIDS patients at Durban's McCord Hospital, was still a young doctor, just starting out at Durban's public R. K. Khan Hospital. He was candid about how little he knew then:

Initially, we began seeing a few cases: young people with strokes. We began seeing people wasting, people with chronic diarrhea, and a few people with myocarditis or with cardiac failure. And in our investigations of these patients, having done everything else, we came to the diagnosis of HIV by exclusion.

Even clinicians with years of professional experience were stymied. Jerry Coovadia, already a seasoned pediatrician at King Edward VIII, recalled that "in 1988 we began to see these kids, and we didn't know how to diagnose them; the serology was there, but for babies it was no good."

Reflecting the pace at which cases emerged in the epidemic's first years, doctors acknowledged into the mid-1990s their difficulty in recognizing AIDS. Baffled by clinical symptoms that should have responded to conventional interventions, they began to discover that the manifestations of HIV disease could take many forms. Lucky Ndokweni, who had trained at the University of Natal and had specialized in orthopedics, struggled to find a diagnosis before he finally identified his first AIDS case in 1993:

That case was a middle-aged male, about 30, who was thrown from pillar to post through all the departments of the hospital. We investigated that person in orthopedics because the presenting complaint was stiffness in the lower back and difficulty in mobility. I never seemed to come up with a reasonable diagnosis. He improved, and we subsequently discharged him, but he came back again. I then decided to take help from my consultant, and we both worked him up. Then, out of the blue, my consultant said, "Why don't we investigate this person for HIV?" And when we investigated, that it was. That it was.

In the large crowded wards of public hospitals, where patients suffering from communicable diseases were common, it was all too easy for doctors to fail to recognize that the typical infectious illnesses they had seen for years were now the consequence of an underlying immune disorder—until ordinary disease patterns changed dramatically. Pinky Ngcakani, now a private practitioner, was a 26-year-old intern in 1994 in Port Elizabeth, an industrial and commercial city in the Eastern Cape, when anomalous cases started to accumulate in the wards. "We would see a lot of ordinary cases, but they were just too bizarre. We'd see a lot of chest infections coming out of nowhere. We knew that TB was endemic, but it was getting out of proportion." As the number of "ordinary" patients with diseases that eluded cure proliferated, Ngcakani and her colleagues began to ask them for consent to test for HIV. To her amazement, about 8 percent of those tested were already positive.

Even those who had begun to develop experience in diagnosing AIDS could still find it difficult. Tugela Ferry, approximately 140 miles northwest of Durban, is a desperately poor, dry, densely populated rural settlement studded with traditional, round, thatched-roofed, single-roomed huts. There, François Eksteen, a devoutly Christian doctor who traces his ancestry to a 1740 Dutch immigrant to South Africa, headed the pediatric services at the Church of Scotland Hospital. Although by 1995 the hospital had already identified a few patients with AIDS, it had not yet faced a full-scale epidemic among its patients. Eksteen knew to be alert to peculiar cases where illnesses proved resistant to treatment.

> You often realize that something more is wrong with the child. It might be marasmus or kwashiorkor, with clinical symptoms that are associated with severe malnutrition, and you realize the child is not responding to the usual approaches. You diagnose tuberculosis, but you realize that this child is not doing well. Eventually we would do the HIV test, and it would come back positive. And regularly what we saw was that the mother was still quite healthy, but the baby was already quite sick.

Having discovered cases of HIV infection in heterosexual men and women and in young children, doctors began to realize that other cases might have passed unnoticed. What meager statistics were assembled by those who first encountered AIDS were almost certainly an undercount. In ruminating on her first HIV case, Glenda Gray concluded, "We probably had been seeing a lot of younger children who died of opportunistic pneumonias which we didn't even think was HIV. We probably had missed a whole lot of the rapid progressors, because we just weren't thinking of it."

Once the flow of patients increased, sooner in some regions than others, doctors began to recognize new cases more readily and became more sensitive to the gravity of their situation. In 1992, Haroon Saloojee, then a 31-year-old politically engaged pediatrician, started his own informal surveillance of newborns at Baragwanath.

> We were suddenly beginning to see more kids dying. Obviously at that stage we weren't doing a lot of testing. It wasn't routine to test every child who potentially had HIV/AIDS. We began to recognize this syndrome: there was this group of children with lymphadenopathy who looked malnourished and obviously had much more serious illnesses than other children. Some of us were already beginning to say that we were not doing enough about this problem.

Epidemic Takeoff

Saloojee was unusual in that he had a sense of foreboding. "There's a doomsday scenario in ten years' time; now is an opportunity." Such concerns were shared by those who had worked abroad and who had come face to face with AIDS in countries already ravaged by the epidemic.

In the first years of the 1980s, Robin Wood, a British-born, Oxford-trained physician who, a decade later, would work at Somerset Hospital with Frank Spracklen treating gay men with AIDS in Cape Town, ran a small clinic in Lusaka, Zambia. At that time, he was responsible as a doctor for "groups participating in game hunting and safaris in the far east of the country, treating crocodile bites and leopard maulings." There, he began to see men dying soon after he diagnosed them with oral candida or wasting syndrome. He and his colleagues tried to make sense of this new phenomenon, in the process following the trajectory of hypotheses proposed by researchers in the United States for what appeared to be a similar disease.

> We would be reading the journals and the information coming out of the States, and we would look at each other and say, "They think it's due to poppers, inhalation of amyl nitrite, by gay men," and we would look at each other and shake our heads and say, "No, that's not right." Next, they thought anal injection of semen was immunosuppressive. Eventually someone put forward that it looked like hepatitis B and was transmitted sexually, and that sounded as though it could be right. But we had no concept of the underlying pathology.

Some years later, in 1987, Clarence Mini, who would return to South Africa only after the apartheid government had lifted the ban on the African National

Congress, was working as a doctor in a hospital in Harare, Zimbabwe, treating the military forces of the ANC. There he was mentored by an Indian professor of medicine with an avid interest in HIV and Kaposi's sarcoma, the cancer that is one of the hallmarks of full-blown AIDS. "He would go around taking biopsies of all these funny skin lesions, and at the time it was something new to us. He was doing research, so he was really forcing all of us who were working there at the time to follow those cases." In addition, Mini and his colleagues were ordered by his professor to test anybody diagnosed with shingles for HIV infection. Testing occurred, of course, in the absence of effective treatment.

In time, Mini began to realize that the wasting he now recognized in Zimbabwe he had previously seen in Lusaka among ANC cadres passing through from military training in Angola to underground warfare in South Africa. There, he had been puzzled by the paradox of significant weight loss and tuberculosis in these well-fed young fighters. With alarm and concern, he concluded these men were viral carriers, bringing the disease with them as they crossed borders.

> We were saying to ourselves, now these guys are in transit, these guys are
> going home, and at some stage, if they are going to meet up with girls,
> this virus is going to spread. When we get home, we would say to ourselves,
> we just have to immerse ourselves in this and not have it devastating
> our country like in Zimbabwe.

A few others, like James McIntyre, already foresaw the epidemic's potential sweep. As a Zimbabwean and a gay man with personal and professional ties to Steven Miller, Dennis Sifris, and others involved in gay HIV treatment and organizations, he was more aware of the epidemic forecasts being made at home and overseas. By the early to mid-1990s, McIntyre recalled, he was predicting that the HIV prevalence rate in South Africa would peak at 30 percent of the population.

> In South Africa at the time, statistical models showed different scenarios
> with condom use, some condom use, no condom use. And it seemed to
> us that the high one was where we were heading, because the rates of
> increase at Baragwanath were absolutely parallel to the projections, and we
> were not seeing any sign that prevention was working.

Henry Sunpath, a deeply religious convert to Christianity from Hinduism, linked the inevitability of a major AIDS epidemic to sexual mores in South Africa. His analysis, in which he also acknowledged the tendency of some to deny the inevitable, was deeply colored by his moral and religious beliefs.

> By the early '90s, AIDS was clearly defined in Africa as heterosexually
> transmitted. So that made it quite clear to us that there is every possibility
> that this is going to grow because of the cultural background of our local

people and the promiscuous lifestyle and the whole system of cohabiting before marriage and multiple partners. We could see it coming and yet, at the same time, with the denial of the government, we wished that it wasn't there.

As the flow of the epidemic began to accelerate, in some places the cases became a fast-moving stream, threatening to swamp the wards. In the first half of the 1990s, Jerry Coovadia, who had displayed no professional or political interest in the gay AIDS epidemic, watched with dismay as the pediatric beds of King Edward VIII Hospital filled with infected children:

It was relentless. It went like a tide, and it just swept through the whole hospital, year by year by year. I remember the doubling time was nine months, a larger and larger proportion of our patients being HIV/AIDS, so that by the mid-1990s or so, 30 to 40 percent of the patients were HIV/AIDS.

By 1997, rural hospitals in KwaZulu-Natal were awash in AIDS. Caroline Armstrong, another devout Christian, a British-born and -trained doctor who moved to South Africa in 1997 when she was 30 years old and who had served in a number of the ex-missionary facilities there, described what greeted her at Murchison Hospital in Port Shepstone, south of Durban.

I just couldn't believe what I was seeing there. Those people, the bulk of the workload was HIV-related. Every time you were on call in the evening, you got people coming in for the first time with major opportunistic infections, who weren't diagnosed, who didn't want to test—there was too much stigma—and you could just see that this was just ravaging the community. It was just unbelievable how many people were HIV positive.

The speed with which the epidemic took off in the Black African population caught many by surprise, despite the dire epidemiological scenarios that had appeared repeatedly in the late 1980s in the *South African Medical Journal*. Pinky Ngcakani had believed, when still a medical student in Durban in the early 1990s, that AIDS was primarily a disease of homosexuals and drug users which "was not as aggressive as it turned out to be." At King Edward VIII Hospital, Raziya Bobat also lacked any sense of foreboding. "I must say that we didn't envisage what happened. It didn't really seem to be a problem that was going to be spread." Her husband, Umesh Lalloo, a pulmonologist who would become head of the Department of Medicine at the Nelson R. Mandela Medical School in Durban, remembered, "I had a junior registrar who came from Zimbabwe, and he told me, 'In five years' time your wards are going to be as full of HIV as in Zimbabwe,' and we said, 'That's not going to happen here.'" His colleague Kogie Naidoo was only somewhat more prescient. She saw AIDS as "important and small. My impression was it was something that could be contained, very much like dysentery and tuberculosis." Looking back in 2004, even Elizabeth Fielder, an English nurse already engaged by the early 1990s in caring for gay men with AIDS in Cape Town, could say: "Never, never, never. I never thought it would ever get like this." In hindsight, Jamila Aboobaker, who had seen her first AIDS case in London in 1984 and her first South African case, a white gay man, a year later, was incredulous at her naiveté. "I didn't expect this epidemic," she said. "I think that was just being stupid. The way the sexual behavior of the population is, it's not surprising. During apartheid, the migrant labor system encouraged promiscuity as wives were not allowed in the cities."

First Cases

Among the doctors who first encountered AIDS cases, it was not uncommon for them to remember their early patients with HIV disease, because of the duration of their encounters, the suffering they witnessed, and the deaths they attended.

For Anisa Mosam, a dermatologist who was at King Edward VIII at the time, "The skin is the window of the body." Her earliest case, in the mid-1990s, offered the most terrible insight into HIV disease.

> The one patient that sticks out very much in my mind was admitted with toxic epidermal necrolysis (TEN); that was basically a drug rash. I think TEN is the nightmare of any dermatologist. It is a condition where you get almost 100 percent stripping of the skin. It's an absolutely horrific thing to look at. TEN has a 90 percent mortality. This patient really just defied all the odds and eventually survived despite this diagnosis.
>
> It was quite a hair-raising experience, because every morning you would walk into the ward, and the more severe patients are kept in the front where the nurses can keep an eye on them. Before you step in, you just pray, "Let his bed not be empty." Because if it is empty, it means he is gone. And you see him there, and then you think, "OK, now pluck up the courage to try and deal with him," because this patient is totally stripped, which means his dermis is showing, he's got blood oozing over him. So it leaves you and the nursing staff exposed to HIV. It was very new to me. I was not as hardened as I am now. You're dealing with your reaction to this patient, and also you want to give this patient the hope that you are not letting this diagnosis affect the way you deal with him.

Kogie Naidoo was in her mid-20s when she worked on the pediatric ward of the same hospital. She recalled with sorrow a little girl she had cared for on the wards.

The one that upset me deeply was about five; she was in the ward because she had developed an HIV-associated lymphoma. I was there daily, giving her a drip and basically seeing to her needs. There were days when she used to follow me around, pass me the swabs. She was just my companion. Wherever I went, she was near; you just needed to look around, she would be sitting in a corner.

I am Hindu speaking, so I normally wear a red dot. When you are married, you are supposed to assume greater vision and knowledge, so the red dot is the symbol of the third eye. In the ward, the kids were given an apple, and the apples all had a little round sticker. So this little one used to put a sticker in the middle of her forehead to emulate me. She was initially very well, and she became sicker and sicker. After six or eight weeks, she eventually died. I can say that now, but could not then. I was called to the ward because the nurses could see no movement. I had seen her early in the day and we were laughing and joking and chatting, and she was talking about her grandmother. Both her parents had died. Her grandmother lived very far away and could not visit her often. She was talking about her grandmother's next visit, and I was teasing her that she was going to stop helping me because she was going home. I couldn't deal with the fact that this child died with AIDS, and she died alone.

She died innocently. She never understood that her parents were infected and she was infected as a result of this. That all of those needles, the chemo, the blown veins, the thrombosed veins, the pain, just injecting her repeatedly, just was for nothing at the end of the day. You are left thinking, "I don't want to really get close to another patient and watch them die."

On occasion, doctors remembered young patients, like Naidoo's, who, by force of circumstance—poverty, abandonment—became boarders in the hospitals to which they had been sent. François Eksteen had a recollection of a young boy at the Church of Scotland Hospital, who was ironically named Nonhlanhla, or "good fortune."

He was brought in by his grandmother in a terribly sick condition. He was about two years old; he had severe kwashiorkor and septicemia and also tuberculosis. After a couple of weeks he slowly started to improve. In the beginning, like many of the children, he was very apathetic and irritable. He started to smile and socialize. His grandmother never came back. The father had brought the child from Durban to his mother. She realized that the child was dying, and she brought him to the hospital. The father came to visit the child one or two times, but basically the father had no social support himself. As often happens in our very unstable times, the mother had just disappeared. They weren't married. This child stayed with us in the hospital up to a year. Now and again, he would get an opportunistic infection, and he would come right again. He was never a very strong child, but in the end he was responding; he would walk in the wards and play a bit with the other children. Sometimes he would come to us and put his arms around our legs. Eventually he died.

Death was a defining feature of these first encounters with AIDS. All involved painful memories. But some seem especially difficult to move on from. Bernhard Gaede was in Durban completing his medical internship at McCord Hospital in 1995 when he began to treat a pregnant woman wracked with opportunistic infections secondary to HIV. Watching the woman and her fetus die almost simultaneously was an agonizing experience.

She had TB; she probably had *Pneumocystis carinii* pneumonia. She was emaciated and she had candida that wasn't responding to treatment. She was really quite ill, and she was about five months' pregnant. I remember having discussions with a number of people around what we should do. It was clear that the baby was still completely unviable. But, especially in her skeletal stage, there was this bulge in her belly, and you could see the fetal movement because she was so thin. I remember just being acutely aware of how unfair this is, just how crazy this disease is; it was just so indiscriminant. She died whilst I was still in the ward, and I really struggled with her dying. It brought up a lot of emotions in me. It wasn't easy to engage with it. This child was going to die in the uterus while the mother was fading away. There was this life that was growing and this body that was dying.

The recollection of a death also tied Bongani Thembela, trained at the University of Natal and King Edward VIII Hospital, to his first AIDS case.

In 1993, I was in private practice in northern Natal, and I had my first AIDS patient there. We struggled with the patient, we struggled with the diagnosis—initially we didn't think about AIDS. Eventually, when he was really dying, the parents phoned me. Now we had discussed with him that when the time comes, he doesn't want to be in hospital; he wants to die at home. So I decided to go and stay with him, go to his house. When I came there, I could see he could die any minute. So I said, "Look, I'll sit with him." So I sat with him, held his hand. We sat there an hour, two hours, three hours, four hours, five hours. Eventually, it was 4:00 in the morning and I had my practice waiting at 7:30, and he died at 4:30. It just took too much out of me, not just the hours—I could recover from that—but the emotional thing was just too much for me.

Coming to AIDS

In time, the dimensions of the South African AIDS epidemic would touch every element of the country's health care system, although the vast majority of cases would fall most heavily on the public sector's hospitals and clinics. But, at the outset, there were choices to be made about how invested individual doctors and nurses would become in caring for those with AIDS. Many did everything possible to avoid the new disease; others simply accepted the unfolding medical challenge and its demands. Very different were those who felt drawn to people sickened by HIV.

The unusual clinical picture presented by their patients became a source of interest and fascination to some doctors. AIDS awakened a sense of scientific excitement, even as the misery of those who were sick underscored the limits of their capacity to intervene. James Muller, who began to serve as the head of the Department of Medicine for Pietermaritzburg's three hospitals in 1994 when he was 45 years old, spoke of coming to grips with a new burden.

> Some things just get thrust upon you. There was no one else to do it. It was
> obviously going to become a major part of the practice of the department,
> so I thought I had to take responsibility for it. Also it was interesting.
> We were learning, learning as we went along. There were new problems to
> be solved, new clinical manifestations to be recognized; the best way is
> to respond to them. It was very unfortunate for the patient, but for the
> clinicians it was fascinating.

Fascination could sustain the drive to understand the pattern of opportunistic infections in AIDS patients and to unravel the complexity of the diagnostic challenges posed by HIV. But it could not long serve to mask the suffering and the inevitability of death in those increasingly filling the medical wards. At King Edward VIII, Umesh Lalloo recalled the mix of professional excitement and clinical despair that would define his early engagement with the epidemic.

> You worked in the medical ward, and the number of cases was beginning
> to increase. It was a challenge to read about AIDS in the literature and
> begin to see these cases. It aroused your own interest, and we used to
> regularly present these patients. We had numerous clinical forums. It was
> the clinical challenge that first attracted me.
> I went through a phase where we were searching for these opportunistic
> infections, identifying HIV infection, treating it. It felt very good, because
> here, as a physician, suddenly you were learning this new type of medi-
> cine, you were getting good at it, and people looked upon you as a leader. If
> you got a patient with TB or pulmonary infiltrate, what do you do? You
> come to see me and I say, "OK, let's do the bronchoscopy for you. Let's
> biopsy this; let's aspirate a node." It became very interesting. But then when

cases started increasing and you didn't have access to all the treatment for opportunistic infections, you watched your patients die. Then, for a year or two, I went through the phase where I said, "Is this worth it?"

Despite the clinical challenge of managing AIDS patients, a few doctors opposed the prevailing view that such cases demonstrated the futility of what medicine could offer under the conditions current in South Africa. Aware of strides that had already been made in treating opportunistic infections in Europe and the United States, they sought to apply these interventions to their own very sick patients. Leon Levin, born in 1963, was drawn to such prospects in his care for children in the years he worked at Johannesburg Hospital, in the mid-1990s.

People had the attitude, "It's only HIV; there's nothing we can do. Just ignore it, and just give them Bactrim." But I began to see that there was more to it than just these children with no [good] prognosis. I began to get a glimmer of hope; with good care, good nutrition, PCP prophylaxis, these children's lives were improved. There was no question that I felt there was something to be done. I grew because the more I got involved, the more I saw what could be done; the more I saw, the more I did, even finding ingenious ways of doing it. It wasn't all doom and gloom.

But, for others, it was precisely the severity of the emerging epidemic, the extent of the suffering, and the profound stigma that those who were sick were compelled to bear that provided the moral foundation for their newfound commitment. Kogie Naidoo, whose apartheid era childhood in Chatsworth—one of the segregated areas of Durban where Indians were compelled to live—had left a lasting impression, said:

I think that the stigma of HIV is what attracted me. The fact that there was clearly such a lack of understanding in our community of how a person gets HIV infected, and the profile of an infected person, and the fact that most people didn't want to be involved without even getting to understand what's going on, is what made me want to stay. I needed to do this for patients and for myself.

Like Naidoo, Neil McKerrow, at Pietermaritzburg's Edendale Hospital, felt touched by the suffering and stigma of those with AIDS. As a pediatrician, he had involved himself with children who had been sexually abused. Now, his interest was in the children who would be compelled to take on adult responsibilities as their mothers' health failed, children who would ultimately be orphaned.

Some of those children will be infected, so by default I became actively involved in caring for infected children. The other default was [that] no other pediatricians were willing to look at that issue. They found it a little too depressing. They found it very demotivating, demoralizing, and they also had a very fatalistic approach. So, they washed their hands of the infants.

The powerful influence of religious commitment, so often at the root of moralistic contempt for those with AIDS, also shaped a compassionate response to the emerging epidemic. For Henry Sunpath, the vista of suffering that he witnessed while at R. K. Khan in Durban touched him deeply. The sense of Christian duty that defined his world as a physician informed the tableau he painted and drove him to ease the suffering of those with AIDS, who had nowhere to turn.

People used to be coming in on stretchers from all over the outlying areas of Durban, absolutely sick, dehydrated, vomiting, hardly able to breathe. And their entire communities used to be coming along with them. "Please help this person; do something." And there was no mechanism in that hospital to take these patients in, to sort them out medically, to equip them with the knowledge and the means to go back home and take care of themselves. The hospital was so overwhelmed with the numbers of these patients that, at the casualty level itself, the basic minimum was done and they were asked to go back home.

It was devastating. I used to go back home and tell my wife, "I just don't know what to do." That showed me the extent to which I really needed to get involved, because it was just so hopeless, looking at the faces of those people, near death and just looking to you to do something.

Jane Hampton, born in Zimbabwe, felt herself called by Christ to serve those despised by others. At home raising children during the epidemic's first years, it was to the AIDS service that she was drawn on returning to medicine at McCord Hospital in 1997 at the age of 42.

I was quite involved in the churches, telling people about the importance about accepting people who had HIV. We all need to have open hearts to people that are HIV positive. One of the stories from the Gospel that I used was, there was a woman who had committed adultery, and everyone brought her to Jesus. He said, the one of you that hasn't sinned, throw the first stone. That is how we should accept people. Not one of us has not sinned. You have to accept people as they are and love them like that and work from there.

In the mid-1990s, upon the victory of the anti-apartheid movement, South Africa was a nation suffused with the culture of political struggle. Not surprisingly some doctors understood their involvement with AIDS as a reflection of the values and commitments of the broader campaign for democracy and social justice. For Eula Mothibi, a Black doctor often mistaken for a nurse because of her race and sex, AIDS represented an issue she could not turn from because Black women, men, and children were dying. A follower of Steven Biko's black consciousness movement in the 1970s,[1] she was acutely sensitive to the ways in which race and racism continued to shape the world of medicine and was angered by the absence of a concerted response on the part of most members of her profession. "There's this deafening silence amongst the doctors. No one is saying anything about these Black people who are dying, you know? So who's going to look after them? No one was interested."

Saul Johnson was a 30-year-old resident in 1995 when the disjunction between the realities of HIV care at Baragwanath Hospital and his expectations of pediatric medicine forced him to confront his own institution.

> I got a lot of satisfaction working with children. The ability to do a lot of curative medicine with children was the attraction. Of course, that changed with HIV. I come from a more activist background, so I was more inclined to challenge the status quo. There was a moral imperative that we had to do something about this disease. This was clearly the challenge— this was the challenge that we needed to face. We just got on and did it, because nobody else was doing it.

Given the poverty of those who began to fall ill with AIDS-related diseases, it is not surprising that doctors in private practice initially played a relatively small role in providing leadership and generally, when consulted, offered episodic and cursory care. But as the epidemic grew, it was not restricted to the poor. It also included those with employer-sponsored medical insurance, which at first slowly and then, in 2005, as a matter of law extended coverage for AIDS-related treatment.[2] Employees covered by such plans sought medical attention in settings other than the overtaxed outpatient departments of public hospitals or the few HIV clinics that had begun to emerge. There were, for example, experienced private doctors who had developed expertise over the years by taking care of gay men. There were also those who saw in AIDS a potential source of income with a new client base. Like others concerned about the economics of private practice, Ramesh Laloo Bhoola, who had been in a private medical partnership since 1976, recalled how his initial reluctance to treat AIDS in Durban crumbled.

> Initially, I wasn't well informed, so I wasn't treating people with AIDS. But my partner in a Blackish area was seeing a lot of them. And then I felt, he's seeing all these patients; perhaps I should also start seeing them. But initially I wasn't keen to treat them; I was sending them away.

Those doctors who took up the challenge of AIDS thus did so for many reasons. But they came to believe that the expanding epidemic had become a defining feature of medical life in South Africa. This was true, for example, for Tony Moll in rural KwaZulu-Natal, who strongly felt that "doctors can't run from it. It's part of medical life." His views were echoed by Bongani Thembela, whose dissatisfactions with the care he witnessed at overburdened urban hospitals led him to migrate from one setting to another. "You either consciously work in a dedicated clinic for HIV/AIDS or you can consciously try to avoid it. You can't run away from it! They are there. You have to treat them."

Facing a Wall of Resistance

Many did work assiduously to distance themselves from HIV and from those who bore its clinical expression in a succession of debilitating conditions. In fact, the medical community, except for the first doctors and nurses who committed themselves to working with AIDS, expressed an almost oceanic indifference to those patients and exhibited a clinical response sometimes indistinguishable from neglect, even cruelty. It was that gulf that profoundly shaped the experience of both caregivers and their patients in the mid- to late 1990s, as AIDS took hold in South Africa.

A pervasive sense of nihilism framed the outlook of those who sought to shield themselves from the epidemic. An AIDS diagnosis was, for them, tantamount to a death sentence; an extended expenditure of time and effort was hardly justifiable. Often unaware of the extent to which the appropriate management of opportunistic infections could make a significant contribution to the well-being of those afflicted with HIV infection, they focused instead on their inability to confront the underlying viral cause of AIDS.

Speaking of the public hospitals in which she had previously worked, Kathryn Mngadi, trained at King Edward VIII and Addington hospitals, said:

> The general mindset of medical practitioners was that there's nothing
> we can do, and patients, once they were diagnosed as being HIV positive, were told, "Well, you must go home." If they came back, they would
> be given whatever, and then you had to go home. They were very seldom admitted.

In 2004, from the vantage point of her position at a hospital run by the Anglo-Gold Corporation for the mining community of Orkney, about 100 miles from Johannesburg, she spoke of a physician whose sense of futility had ultimately driven him from South Africa.

> There's a doctor who was here who's now left to work in Canada. Oddly
> enough, he would encourage people to be tested. He would really work
> them up medically to the very last, but he had a penchant for writing big on
> the file "AIDS." Then he would say to me, "Why do you even bother? What

is the point?" I'd give presentations on what we were doing at the clinic, and he'd say, "Oh, but they're dying anyway!" And it never really changed. I think it's part of the reason he left, because, as he put it, "Everywhere I turn there's just HIV, HIV. When I became a doctor, I was looking at rheumatoid arthritis, hypertension, diabetes; and now everything is just HIV. I'm so sick of it."

Those whose work, even under the economic limits of public hospital care, had been suffused with enthusiasm about effective clinical medicine voiced dismay about the changes they were seeing. Andrew Ross, who spent the 1990s caring for patients at Mosvold Hospital in rural KwaZulu-Natal, about 250 miles from Durban, spoke in emotionally measured tones about the clinical impotence he and his colleagues faced: "The impression I got is that doctors find it difficult. You have these chronic diarrhea patients who are in and out and in and out and not really getting any better." Worse still was the growing number of deaths, especially from previously treatable disorders.

The TB ward has increasingly become a place where people come and die. The TB ward used to be somewhere that patients came, they had TB, but they were relatively well. They were given their medications; they then went home to take their medications. Now, what we are finding is that people come to the TB ward, and then they stay a long time and then they die. Or they go home and take their medications and then come back to the hospital to die.

It was the transition from effective medicine to clinical impotence that most impressed Jerry Coovadia, a professor of pediatrics with years of experience.

Clinical medicine had always been my passion. There is no equivalent thrill to being on intake, seeing a seriously ill patient, and you are the first person making an accurate diagnosis and treating. It was a part of my life which was just absolutely great, and I wanted to transmit that excitement to the people who were working with me. That just disappeared with the AIDS epidemic; it just killed it. From about the mid-90s, it just destroyed our excitement and our enthusiasm about clinical medicine, because the problems are so uniform. Clinical medicine, the exciting part of it and the critical part of it, depends on the diversity of problems you see. That just goes out if everything is AIDS, because everything is thrush and everything is the same type of pneumonia and everything is malnutrition. And it just becomes a grey pall of despair.

A sense of futility could serve to justify barring patients from already overburdened hospitals. This seemed utterly cruel to those who believed that people with AIDS needed and deserved care, and it provoked a sense of outrage. Jeanne Dixon, a nurse with experience as an educator and administrator, had come as a volunteer to Grey's Hospital in Pietermaritzburg, on whose board she served, to help staff an AIDS clinic. She described two encounters that fueled her resentment.

> It was painful. I had a patient who was too weak to walk. We didn't have a bed for her. I knew that the person who brought the young woman here was going to have to put her in a taxi, and when they got to the other side, carry her little body halfway up a mountain somewhere. Just to lie there, in pain, unattended, dehydrated. On another occasion, a 42-year-old man, who was critically ill, was brought to the hospital from a rural area by his 10-year-old grandson. I requested of the casualty officer that the patient be admitted overnight as he was in no condition to undertake a long taxi journey and because it was expecting just too much of a 10-year-old to shoulder the responsibility of accompanying his dying grandfather home. After much begging and explaining, the doctor said: "I'm not going to admit him!" I eventually put the patient on a trolley. He died two hours later, parked in a passage with that little boy at his side.

Given the sheer magnitude of AIDS cases, ever-increasing numbers of patients did, however, gain entry to hospitals. But, once admitted, they often experienced a pattern of neglect. In her first year in South Africa, Caroline Armstrong found work, among other places, in a 1,000-bed rural hospital in KwaZulu-Natal.

> It was there that I first started to see what was going on in Africa with HIV. There was no real investigation and management of the opportunistic infections. They were just written off, because nobody knew what to do with them. So people weren't looking for cryptococcal meningitis; they couldn't treat it anyway. They weren't looking for opportunistic parasites in the stool. HIV was there. It was known to be quite a big problem in the medical wards, but it was ignored, and people were written off.

Once he became chief of medicine at King Edward VIII, Umesh Lalloo was forced to reflect upon his own therapeutic nihilism because of the impact it had on patients and younger doctors.

> What I began to see happening around me was a sense of hopelessness developing, not only amongst the patients but amongst the medical staff. I sensed in the minds of the junior doctors, they were beginning to question what the hell are they doing here. If 80 percent of your patients have AIDS and you can't do anything, what am I as a doctor?

What really turned me around was one incident, where I was doing rounds with my team and we came to one patient. We discussed his cardiac problem, discussed treatment, spoke to the patient, outlined to him what his problem was. When I saw the next patient, I knew he had advanced AIDS. There was nothing you could do, and we skipped him. I understand Zulu. That patient told the patient next to him, "I wonder why the doctor doesn't want to see me today; I think I am going to die." I heard this and I sort of froze in my tracks. I suddenly realized that the patient is right; this is the message I sent out to him.

The impact of the ethos of clinical limits on doctors was underscored by Dalu Ndiweni, who had immigrated to South Africa from Zimbabwe in 2002, at age 45. He noted how radically different the response was to hospitalized infected and uninfected children.

Young doctors felt, if this is the way it's going to go, then there's no future in medicine. You could see their response when a patient was HIV negative. For this child, you must do everything, because he's negative. This one you must save. It was an expression of joy; there was good reason why we should succeed. Here, there was a future.

So intense could be the resistance to treating those with HIV that even an unfounded suspicion could provide the warrant for medical neglect. Andrew Ross described an occasion when physicians simply refused to accept the laboratory evidence with which they were presented.

For a lot of the patients who are HIV positive, the doctors in fact stop thinking. You've got AIDS, and you are going to die. If you've got any other illness except TB, well, we won't investigate you because it's all part of the AIDS problem. So we don't really understand what's wrong with you, but you are HIV positive, and we can't do anything. We just provide nursing care for you. There is one patient that is in fact HIV negative, has been tested twice, but the doctor's convinced that the test is wrong. She's been labeled as positive although her two tests have made her negative, and she hasn't been investigated and she has developed gangrene. She still hasn't been investigated, and she is going to die.

"There were doctors," said Salome Charalambous, referring to her experience treating miners for the AngloGold Corporation, "who would write on the patient's notes, 'advanced HIV disease. Not for CPR.' And they had no basis to say 'advanced,' just because the patient had lost weight or something like that. That gave the nurses almost the passport or right to ignore the patient."

Nihilism transformed AIDS into something unworthy of attention, uninteresting. Obstetrician James McIntyre recalled the way in which infected women who had delivered babies at Baragwanath were treated in the early 1990s. In this case, the neglect had mortal consequences.

It was the stage when everybody was completely terrified by HIV, nursing staff, everybody. Women, if they were known to be HIV positive initially, had bright orange biohazard stickers on their files, and they were put at the far end of the labor room. In 1991, I was very concerned because I really felt that these women were not being treated as they should be. Two of them died really through neglect, one from a postpartum hemorrhage that nobody wanted to sort out; one because she was put far away from other laboring mothers and not monitored properly. There was another woman who had Kaposi's of the throat who died in labor because the anesthetists wouldn't look after her.

At Baragwanath Hospital, Saul Johnson saw the pediatric services overwhelmed by the confluence of rural migration into Johannesburg and the decision of the new ANC government in 1994 to provide free health care to children under five.[3] With HIV disease adding to the crowded wards, he pressed his colleagues to investigate the disorders of children with AIDS, to no avail.

There was no research being done. I raised this, and I didn't get a very positive response. I said, "What's going on in these kids? We don't know if we're getting PCP in South Africa. There's very little written about PCP in developing countries. We know it's very common—it occurs everywhere—but is that what these kids have got? Then we need to treat them more actively and find out." I couldn't interest any of the senior academics in finding out what was behind this lung disease. It went from being quite exotic to suddenly being overwhelming.

Johnson's memory was echoed by Leon Levin. Because Baragwanath, where he was trained, is a teaching hospital affiliated with Witwatersrand's medical school, its doctors would have been among the most clinically sophisticated in South Africa. But with the rise in AIDS, the response of these doctors was striking. They too, according to Levin, increasingly refused to become involved.

At Baragwanath, they are treating extremely ill children. By the time they get to Baragwanath, they are extremely ill, and the children with HIV are certainly not alone. There are other children there that were dying with severe diseases. So in the beginning—because the numbers were small—you did your best for everybody. It was unbelievable. You could see the progression of the epidemic to the degree that people were really hard on the disease. I suppose one can understand; it's extremely hard to see children dying. It's extremely hard to be helpless. I can understand people's reaction, but it's really hard to see not only what was happening to the children, but what was happening to colleagues.

Haroon Saloojee, Levin's colleague at Baragwanath Hospital, recalled how even the deaths of children became so routine that careful investigation seemed unnecessary.

Our initial response was, I suppose, curiosity and interest, like always. Saying OK, so this is what HIV/AIDS is like, it's a learning curve. Finding these fascinating new diseases, how children were behaving differently. There came a stage where we began to notice that there were a lot of these kids out there, and they do die. We have a tradition of monthly audits of deaths. I remember that phenomenon, where we discussed each case that died in all the different wards at Baragwanath and went through case by case. We got to the stage when we said, "OK, we had six deaths in the wards this month, three were HIV deaths and three non-HIV." The three non-HIV cases we would go through, discussing what they have died of. The three HIV deaths, it was felt like we got to the stage where it was nothing unusual. There was no point. Let's discuss the more interesting deaths.

Even when research began to show the prospect of making a significant impact on the clinical course of AIDS, resistance remained. Mark Cotton, a pediatrician, had trained for five years in the United States to become expert on issues surrounding pediatric AIDS. In 1996, at age 40, he returned to Tygerberg, a public hospital in Cape Town, aware of the studies in the United States that had demonstrated the possibility of radically reducing the rate of HIV transmission from infected women to their newborns. Anxious to see how such research findings could be brought to bear on the problem of AIDS in children in South Africa, he met a wall of resistance.

Our obstetric department is seen as the most academically productive department in the faculty. It produced more Ph.D.'s than any other department; its publication record is the best. It had a Medical Research Council–funded perinatal unit for about 10 to 15 years. The HIV prevalence had gone up from less than 1 percent in the Western Cape to 4 percent. But the department wasn't interested, not at all. They were not interested in changing their established approach. Some people felt: what's the point of preventing HIV in the kids, when the parents were all going to die? Why even admit the parents? Let them all die.

He ultimately came to the conclusion that it was not simply bureaucratic inertia that was blocking his way at Tygerberg, an Afrikaner-dominated institution which is among the largest hospitals in South Africa. "I think there is a very strong religious influence, and a very Calvinistic influence. It was the idea that the people were being promiscuous, and they got their desserts."

Finally, the pressure on hospital beds, the sense of futility, and the need to make room for patients with better prospects could lead doctors to discharge patients in a way that all but consigned them to death. Saul Johnson effectively fought one such effort at Baragwanath Hospital, fully aware that there were many others about whom he knew nothing.

> There were times when medical registrars would just discharge our pa-
> tients, and these were young women. I remember one case very vividly. This
> woman had chronic illness, fever, and was just generally very weak and
> unable to walk. I worked her up for TB, no TB. But then the investigation
> seemed to stop. She was just written off, given antibiotics, and I heard that
> this one patient of ours had been discharged; and I went to see her, and
> her condition had not improved. So I phoned up the medical registrar and
> I said, "Why have you discharged our patient? She clearly is not better."
> And his point of view was, "Well, there's nothing more we can do. She's an
> AIDS patient. We've done so many investigations, can't really find anything
> wrong, she must just go home to her family now." He didn't quite say
> "go home and die," but that was the implication of what he was saying.

The sense of futility and indifference that doctors and nurses encountered in clinical settings had a dramatic impact on medical education. Medical students, if they heard of AIDS at all, learned to discount it. For Themba Mabaso, who attended the University of Natal in the 1980s and who was the son of one of the few Black doctors trained under apartheid, AIDS was a disease of other countries, found in West Africa and the United States. Farida Amod, also at Natal at that time, learned about HIV as "the tenth cause of something. So, if there was any case you presented, and somebody said, 'And what else can cause this?' as a last resort you would say 'HIV.'"

Instructors focused on and taught the treatment of the chronic noninfectious diseases, ignoring HIV/AIDS. Amod recalled, "The cases we were exposed to were the general medical cases, hypertension, strokes, diabetes. I don't remember ever presenting a case of HIV or having that in my exams." Those studying at the University of the Witwatersrand Medical School in Johannesburg a few years later had similar experiences. As one reported, "Faculty were into teaching us cardiology and pulmonology and renal disease; to the physicians of the time, those were the interesting cases. The HIV cases were just patients who got an infection."

When the importance of AIDS was not denied, students were led to believe that treatment was futile. Liesl Page-Shipp, an AIDS doctor and researcher working for the Aurum Institute for Health Research in 2004, recalled that for most teachers at "Wits," "HIV was regarded as completely untreatable, to the point that I came out thinking it wasn't worth doing a lumbar puncture on a person; it's unbelievable now." When Pinky Ngcakani was a medical student, also in the early 1990s, her instructors drew a "dark and gloomy" clinical picture of AIDS. More ominously, "when we started getting lectures on HIV, we got to understand it was something that you should avoid at all costs. I mean, that was the message then; I suppose that's the message now too."

Saul Johnson, while at Witwatersrand in the 1980s, was most aware of AIDS "on an intellectual level," especially once he interrupted his medical training to begin a bachelor's of science degree in hematology. As a consequence, he became interested in the burgeoning debate initiated by Peter Duesberg in the United States as to whether the virus, HIV, actually caused AIDS. (This debate would later draw the attention of President Thabo Mbeki, Nelson Mandela's successor.) But AIDS was absent from his clinical training. "From a scientific point of view, I was very interested in the debate, certainly aware of what was happening elsewhere in Africa, but not really seeing it on a visceral level or on a clinical care level." Salome Charalambous, who began at Witwatersrand a few years after Johnson, in the early 1990s, recalled learning little about AIDS beyond its microbiology. "Our virologist was Professor Schoub—he used to run the National Institute of Virology—and he taught us a lot about the virus and its structure. That was basically all they knew at that point."

Fears of Contagion

When they first encountered AIDS, South African doctors and nurses, like their counterparts around the world, feared that they would become infected. Clarence Mini recalled that when he was still in exile with the ANC in Zimbabwe, he was in charge of a district hospital, working very long hours. Because his responsibilities included surgical duties, he was often covered with the blood of patients. Touching meant possible infection, a condition he accepted with both fear and stoic fatalism.

> I was very afraid. When I was doing all these surgeries, I was saying
> to myself, "If any of these people have got AIDS"—and this was like
> swimming in blood—"then God help me." Because needle pricks in sur-
> gical procedures like cesarean sections were common, because you
> could puncture your skin. Sometimes you don't feel it, but when you
> finish, before you take off your gloves, when you looked at the glove, this
> blood is inside the glove. And you say, "Wow." You panic because you
> have punctured the glove, and it is possible that you punctured your
> skin.

He was convinced many times that he had been infected, but refused to test himself. "There was no point because tomorrow I was going to be on duty in the same place. There was no point at the time; it would have meant testing every week."

For many doctors and nurses, the fears expressed by Mini, the possibility of needle stick injuries that might occur when taking blood from patients or when providing injections, became a source of persistent anxiety, especially as the number of patients increased. Harried and rushed, they found that their worst nightmare, needle stick wounds, began to occur with alarming frequency. Sue Roberts, a nurse who established the infection control unit at Helen Joseph Hospital in Johannesburg in the early 1990s, reported, "We have quite a lot of needle stick injuries, and the fact that 60 percent of the ward patients are HIV positive means the chance of getting HIV is much higher than it would be in the United States." Describing the experience of clinicians in the AngloGold mine hospitals, where about 30 percent of the patients were infected, Liesl Page-Shipp estimated that "at any one time in our two hospitals—we have over 30 doctors— one person is on postexposure prophylaxis."

At Baragwanath Hospital in Johannesburg, it was both the press of working in crowded wards and the special challenges posed by care for infants that exposed interns and residents to increased risk, noted Haroon Saloojee, who headed the neonatal unit from the mid- to late 1990s.

> It is difficult taking blood in little babies. It's a very busy service. The danger is that because of the rush, we are often negligent. We all felt that it was much easier putting up intravenous lines without gloves, so we never put on gloves. But because we were so busy, we left needles lying around. The young doctors began to get exposed to these.

For young doctors, taking blood was especially anxiety provoking. Farida Amod, who would go on to care for AIDS patients, recalled that during her training she and her colleagues simply refused to do so.

> When I was an intern, I saw my first patient with AIDS, a patient with an interstitial pneumonia which turned to be *Pneumocystis*. I refused to take her blood, and the residents had to take it. None of the interns wanted to take blood from the patient. I was afraid.

In the early 1990s, there was no prophylaxis available to doctors and nurses who suffered needle stick injuries. When Aresh Misra, born in 1968, experienced his first such exposure during his internship, there was little he could do but carry on.

> I was putting a drip on a patient, and he stuck the needle into my arm. He was drunk and violent. Basically, I squeezed the wound and cleaned it. That

was it. That was all we had at the time. I started doing my HIV test every two months after that. When it was still negative, it was a relief.

The next time he suffered a wound, the picture had changed. Performing a cesarean at Baragwanath, he had access to a single dose of the antiretroviral AZT. It was the first time he learned of the drug. In time, the most sophisticated hospitals had developed protocols for meeting the needs of staff who experienced needle stick injuries. In 1997, when Anisa Mosam, a 29-year-old dermatologist, suffered a wound, King Edward VIII had prophylactic AZT kits available.

> As a registrar, my job was to do biopsies. I remember this lady, she was middle-aged, with quite extensive Kaposi's sarcoma. I was biopsying a lesion on her side, and I pricked myself. In this kind of environment, because of the pressures—the number of AIDS patients we saw in a day in our clinic averaged 50–100—we invariably had needle stick injuries. Because of that, I didn't think it was a big deal; it really didn't affect me.
>
> And I went home and was telling my husband about it. He said, "You must report this, you have to." I was breastfeeding my son at the time. We called in; there was somebody in virology who was in charge of all the needle stick injuries. We reported it, and I had to come down to the matron and get the AZT.

In addition to being placed on medication, she had to terminate breastfeeding her ten-month-old child.

When Felicity Cope, an AIDS nurse at Somerset Hospital in Cape Town, suffered a puncture wound, she knew to demand prophylactic medication.

> It was a busy clinic, and the nursing staff was very depleted. We had a patient who was very sick with a very high viral load and almost no CD4 and dementia. I had taken her blood, and she wouldn't keep her arm still. As I was pulling it out, she pushed my arm, which ripped the needle out sideways, so it was a deep puncture wound with a deep scratch. Her blood was all over her arm, my hands, the outside of the needle, the couch, the bed, the floor. I was 100 percent convinced that I was going to seroconvert, there was very little doubt in my mind. It was just a really bad needle stick injury.
>
> I'm told that I behaved in a very calm manner. I certainly didn't feel in the slightest bit calm. I think I was functioning in automatic. Evidently, I just put my things down and said to the nurse, "Nurse, finish up here," and I walked over calmly to the tap and squeezed my finger and washed my hands with the alcohol, and then walked around the corner to the pharmacy and when I spoke to the pharmacist I was evidently still calm as well.

I said to him, "Please, could I have some AZT and 3TC," and he said, "Who
for?" and I said, "Me, and give it to me now, please." Something on
my face made him say, "Certainly." Maybe he just wasn't going to refuse me
anyway—I don't know whether that was because he knew me, or whether
it was because I looked as if I might kill him if he didn't. I took the old
high dose of AZT and 3TC, and I had very, very bad side effects. The longest
period of my life so far has been the month that I was taking them.

While some were able to take their medication without such side effects,
others, like pediatrician Dalu Ndiweni at Johannesburg Hospital, suffered as had
Cope. The experience left awful memories.

I was actually very sick for the 28 days I took the antiretrovirals. It was a
combination of AZT and 3TC. I slept poorly all the time. I had no energy;
I couldn't do anything. I didn't have an appetite. I don't know whether
it was the drug or the anxiety. But I felt better a week after I stopped taking
the medications.

It was not just the prospect of needle stick wounds that galvanized anxiety.
Even among the doctors and nurses who were committed to caring for patients
with HIV and AIDS, some struggled with ambivalence: dread on one hand,
compassion on the other. Touching, extending their own bodies toward the sick,
often became the act in which that conflict played out. Kogie Naidoo was unusual
in asserting that she was never hampered by such fears.

I have never once held the fear. I felt then and I still feel now that touching
is an essential part of healing. Part of the lack of emotional connection with
most of the adults and children is because nobody wants to touch them
and to love them. Fortunately, for me, I haven't had a single needle stick
injury. I have been fortunate.

More common was the view of Ashraf Coovadia, who had seen his first HIV
patients in Zambia, where he was born and trained. "The fear was always there. It
was a very fearful thing having to deal with AIDS patients."
    While still a relatively young physician caring for a dying patient—a South
Asian man from Malawi—Umesh Lalloo was filled with a mix of contradictory
feelings.

He was seen by private physicians, and they didn't know what was going
on. He had chronic diarrhea, and I said, "Look, you must do an HIV test."
It came back positive. I went into his history, and he belonged to a very
wealthy family in Malawi, and the way he got HIV was through frequenting
brothels. So he told his parents, and his parents phoned their priest in

Pakistan for the priest to guide them. And the priest advised them that the doctor is mad. He doesn't know what he's talking about, and your son doesn't have AIDS. And they discharged him and took him to Pakistan. He came back. As I remember, he had candida; he had several episodes of PCP. We put him on the first antiretroviral drug, AZT, then in large doses, which made him very sick. While that was happening, his wife came in sick; she was vomiting. The children got sick, and they were vomiting. Then he died, his wife died, and, subsequently, his children died.

I remember his family then became very grateful for the support I provided. I must confess, they did send me a gift of nuts, and I was a bit wary of touching them. I don't know why, but it was kind of an early experience. You are not sure what this disease was all about, and somehow felt that they were contaminated. I told myself that is sheer stupidity, and I made a point of eating them. I felt guilty to have had those thoughts.

Tony Moll, a veteran doctor and hospital administrator in Tugela Ferry who would develop a remarkable program for people with AIDS, including home care and hospice services, recoiled from physical contact with his first HIV patient.

She was already in her early 40s, but she looked well and healthy, and she didn't even need admission. But I could say that we were afraid to touch her, although we did examine her. You had the fear that here was something not well understood that you were dealing with. And as a doctor, it creates some fear, even though by that time it was well documented that you couldn't get it by touching.

Looking back on his own early experience, Dalu Ndiweni spoke self-mockingly about the precautions he had felt compelled to take and about the context within which he had acted.

One of the first cases I saw was a patient who had Kaposi's. Most of those patients were put in different cubicles. We all put masks, put gowns on there, and you were also terrified to go in there. That always amuses me in a sad kind of way; it was a lack of understanding. We could not really get HIV in that way. Kaposi's was not going to jump out of this guy and bite my nose.

Although many nurses, like doctors, sought to avoid contact with AIDS patients, they had less freedom to do so. Consequently, they used whatever precautions were available to them. Veliswa Labatala, an ANC stalwart raised in the 1980s in Khayelitsha, when it served as a site of anti-apartheid militancy, revealed, with some hesitation, an episode that occurred during her training as a nurse in the late 1990s when she was in her early 20s.

When I was doing my midwifery in the labor wards, I remember one lady came, very, very thin, and she'd never attended antenatal clinic. The first thing the sister in charge of that labor ward said was, "High risk!" and high risk then meant HIV. "Double up your gloves!" And then we had to take some bloods, and then we asked for an HIV test. What was interesting, we diagnosed AIDS before doing the blood test. She stayed in the postnatal ward for a week, and the result came back negative. Isn't that interesting? Just tells the attitude we had. We all reacted negatively.

Helga Holst, with years of primary care experience in rural settings, had come to South Africa in 1978 when she was 26 years old. Now the superintendent of the private, but government-subsidized, McCord Hospital where she trained, she remembered that in the mid-1990s, among her nurses, "aprons were worn, boots were worn or overshoes if you were dealing with a patient who had diarrhea; even now in 2004, the nurses wear gloves when they change the bed sheets." A devout Christian dedicated to developing sensitive and professional services for HIV-infected individuals, she recognized the sources of anxiety in her staff.

The fear is really significant, and it's a fear which has two prongs. One is the fear, because our nurses are female, is my partner, my husband, my boyfriend unfaithful? Have I caught this already? This isn't talked about openly. And then, can I catch it from my patients? These two fears, and looking after young people their own age, or like their sisters, or their mothers, or their fathers, who are dying in front of them. At the same time, a funeral of a relative or a friend who they know, every Saturday—and now it's not just every Saturday.

When fear and anger joined ignorance, the results could be ugly. Eric Goemaere, a Belgian-trained tropical disease specialist, had set up an AIDS clinic under the auspices of Doctors without Borders (Médecins sans Frontières, or MSF) in the township of Khayelitsha on the sand flats outside Cape Town. As late as 1999, there were

terrible stories of women who were shouted at when they were HIV positive. I remember one that came here to complain. She was delivering, and the nurses started to point a finger and said, "If I get that disease from you, I am going to catch you, and now you are going to clean your placenta yourself, and I don't touch you." So the women were forced to clean their placenta.

Stigma

Stigma provided the final building block for the edifice of neglect. Touching those infected with HIV was all the more difficult because the disorder carried a moral taint. To have the virus was, for many, to be guilty of bad behavior, of having corrupted oneself, or of having been contaminated by others. Kathryn Mngadi, in 2004 the medical director of AngloGold's AIDS program in Orkney, bluntly stated:

> In South Africa, sexuality itself is something that's hardly spoken about. When you're diagnosed as HIV positive, nine out of ten South Africans will think you are promiscuous. They make an exception for people who have been raped, but other than that, you are promiscuous. That is the beginning and the end of it, and you got what you deserved. Their behavior may be exactly the same as your behavior, but because they don't have that infection or they haven't tested or gotten sick yet, you got what you deserved. It's odd; in a mining environment, if you have a lot of girlfriends, a lot of sexual partners, it's a very macho thing, but if you get HIV, then you're getting what you deserved. It's not quite congruent, but there it is.

Even children could be stigmatized because they bore the sins of their parents. Dalu Ndiweni said the attitude of his colleagues to the babies he saw was, "Mom and dad behaved so badly."

While many bore the experience of stigma in silence, some could react with outrage. In Durban, at the AIDS clinic at King Edward VIII Hospital, Sister Gabi Mbanjwa used her professional training and good sense to soothe a hostile patient, pressing him to reveal the reason for his anger.

> He was 23 years old. He was very, very violent. He didn't want to talk about anything related to HIV/AIDS. He wanted treatment, and that's it. So I said, "Excuse me, I would like to talk to you. Let's go to the consulting room." When we got to the consulting room, I held the hand of that patient, and I asked the patient to look at my eyes. I said, "Just tell me what it is that makes you behave like this, because your behavior is not acceptable at all. Just tell me, and feel free, what is it that worries you?" The patient said, "You know what? I only have one girlfriend, and this girlfriend said to me that I'm her first boyfriend. Now when I went to the private doctor, he told me that I'm HIV positive because I've been sleeping around, which is something I've never done." I said, "OK, I'm sorry for that doctor, because he said something bad to you. Sometimes we, as health care workers, do make mistakes, because we are human beings like everybody. I am saying just on behalf of him, 'Sorry.'"

While many physicians avoided direct confrontations with colleagues who gave voice to such stigmatizing attitudes, some did not. Gary Maartens, head of the clinical infectious disease unit and founder of the HIV clinic at Cape Town's premier public hospital, Groote Schuur, learned to forcefully correct his peers.

People are a bit more careful about coming out with it now than they used to be, but I think people do see this in some crazy way as God's punishment for being sinful. Usually when I encounter it, it's in a setting where I have got the microphone. Whenever I become aware of it in that setting, it's easy to demolish that view: "That is a judgmental view, which has no place in medicine." It's easily recognized as such by the audience, so usually it's quite easy to deal with. With the students, I am quite explicit. I give an example: here, you have got a nurse who was injured in the course of her duties, and she is HIV positive; here, you have got a child, and here you've got a gay prostitute. Who do you treat? It's amazing how many of them gravitate towards "the innocent" as opposed to "the guilty." I try and point out to students that you can't have innocent or guilty patients, just sick and sicker patients.

Medical institutions not only failed to provide a protective shield against such attitudes, they commonly reproduced them. It was not simply white doctors who held such views. Paul Kocheleff, a Belgian-born doctor who first encountered AIDS in Burundi when he was 38 years old and who would establish AIDS clinics at both Edendale and Grey's hospitals in the late 1990s in Pietermaritzburg, reported that his white medical colleagues would say, "Oh these people, the Black people, they behave like animals in their sexual activity." But Black nurses could also embrace stigmatizing attitudes. He recalled that he had asked a nurse to hold a baby while he examined the child's mother, who had AIDS. The nurse placed the baby on the floor, refusing to keep it in her arms.

The extent to which neglect could be carried appalled Sister Margaret Shangase, a 62-year-old Black nurse who worked at Edendale Hospital before retiring and who had witnessed wards where AIDS patients could be found soiled by waste and vomit.

I used to take rounds whenever I had a chance. I would find patients lying, not being cleaned. And when I asked the sisters, they said, "No, we're too busy." Some said, "No, we have no protective material. We couldn't attend him without protective material, because we are going to contract the virus." People were scared. One day, I even told them, "It is really bad to watch what you are doing. One day, you will be lying here. And how would you feel if we neglected you like this? And unfortunately, some of you are already HIV positive, but you do not know. So good people, treat these patients. They are just patients like any other patients. One day, your daughter will be lying here with AIDS."

Jerry Coovadia, professor of pediatrics at the Nelson Mandela School of Medicine, whose youth and early professional life was shaped by the anti-apartheid movement, was even sharper in his judgment of the nurses at King Edward VIII Hospital.

> The nurses were often tied up with their own views on HIV and stigma and discrimination, so they were probably worse than us doctors. I am talking about [Black] African nurses. How they treated the mothers was a reflection of what was going on in the communities, a total denial of the epidemic, and discrimination against people who are HIV infected. The nurses here can be a particularly obdurate and a very conservative element.

Such attitudes persisted at Baragwanath Hospital as late as 2004, James McIntyre noted. "I think there still was and to some extent remains, a judgmental attitude amongst nurses, especially in obstetrics. You know, you are killing your babies because you slept around. Why are you putting us at risk?"

Administrative Hostility

The pattern of hostility and indifference among health care workers—both doctors and nurses—existed within an administrative culture that not only permitted but reinforced such attitudes. That it was now Black men, women, and children who were in need, rather than the gay white men of the earlier AIDS epidemic, made no difference. To be sure, there were exceptions: hospital managers who saw in AIDS a crisis that required special commitments, departments that welcomed the innovative work of doctors who took on the new heterosexual epidemic. But bureaucratic rigidity, fiscal constraints, and the pervasive stigma that informed the response to HIV provided fertile ground for practices and policies that made the work of caregivers obstacle-ridden.

When he arrived in Pietermaritzburg in 1996, Paul Kocheleff was struck by the absence of any concerted effort to organize AIDS-related services.

> What was the activity for the problem of HIV? There was nothing, there was absolutely nothing. In Pietermaritzburg, you have three hospitals. These three hospitals are the reflection of the apartheid period. The biggest one, for the Black community, is called Edendale Hospital. It's there that I got my position initially. The other one is called Grey's. That was the hospital for the white people. And then you had Northdale Hospital, the hospital for the Indian people. I knew that in Northdale Hospital, there was absolutely no HIV clinic. There was no HIV clinic in Grey's Hospital. In Edendale, there was a Romanian lady who tried to do something, something with nothing.
> "Nothing" means that nobody was interested in what she was doing. Nobody was supporting her. Nobody was giving her some help or an

opinion of what to do. The venue she was working in was absolutely
terrible. Not only was it terrible because it was small, but it was also not a
venue for HIV. On Monday afternoons, she had the place. The other days,
it was for neurology and other consultations. And if the people of neurology were busy on Monday afternoon, she just had to go someplace else.
So, she had no place.

Jeanne Dixon recalled the administrators at Grey's who freely gave voice to
their prejudices, making mocking and contemptuous remarks about her work.
These reactions were all the more striking, given her role on the hospital's board.

A very senior member of the hospital once said to me, "I can cure all your
problems, my dear. All I need is a shotgun." And you know, that might
have been perceived to be a bit of a joke, a bit funny, but it spoke deeply to
me about how she really felt. Later, I was lobbying for mother-to-child
intervention. And she came, as I climbed into my car one evening, and she
leaned against the bonnet, and she said, "So you're into saving orphans
now, are you?"

Margaret Shangase described how managerial truculence made her efforts so
difficult.

Sometimes I wanted to do things, and the management would not understand. It helps a lot, for instance, that we have events, especially in rural
areas, because they do not have access to TV, and some don't even have
access to radios. So I would ask the staff at the AIDS unit to go to one of the
schools or to a certain hall in the rural area and give awareness to those
people. And I would ask for orange juice and some biscuits or some
sandwiches. I knew that was going to motivate people to attend, because
some of them used to walk long distances. The hospital refused. I think it
was lack of understanding, because when we were talking about AIDS, you
could see that we were talking Greek to some of them.

In Johannesburg, a leading academic physician proposed to Ian Sanne, who
had assumed a leadership role in HIV clinical trials, that the treatment of AIDS be
moved from his hospital. Indeed, so anxious was he to accomplish this goal that he
made what in other circumstances might have been viewed as a generous offer.

My chief specialist, the head of the Department of Internal Medicine, was
still trying to shift HIV out of the academic hospital. They literally wanted
to give me a ward in a hospital that had been closed, a 200-bed ward. At
the time, I refused to take it, because I thought, "They are trying to dump
the HIV problem onto somebody outside; it's not our problem." While

I think it would have been quite nice to have a 200-bed hospital, in retrospect I think it was the right move. It had to stay a problem for everyone.

At Baragwanath Hospital, where Tammy Meyers was determined to create a clinic for children with AIDS, the administration made it clear that she could expect no support from them. They said, " 'You can do it if you want to do it, but don't expect any kind of assistance from us.' There were one or two people on the staff that were interested and would help out occasionally, but it was really on my shoulders." When, two years later, the opportunity presented itself for her to visit the United States for a three-month training sabbatical, the administrators were true to their word.

> Before I went overseas in 1998, I said, "I'm going away. Is there not anybody that can be allocated to assist at the clinic?" The response was, "No, you wanted the clinic. It was your baby. Now you're going away, don't expect anything from us."

And, during her period away, the clinic, without staffing, languished. When she returned with new expertise in HIV care, she could still garner neither collegial nor material support.

> When I came back and had the intention of working with children with HIV, no one else was interested in doing it. Everyone felt overburdened with what they were doing. There also had been ongoing budgetary cuts for the last 15 years. Patients were being sent elsewhere. They were doing whatever they could not to have children with HIV here. So I said, "OK. I would like to start an AIDS clinic." Our pediatric clinic was on the third floor. There was no space, there were no rooms, and no one was going to give space to have a clinic. That was it. It was very difficult.

Like Meyers, Mark Cotton, in Cape Town, who had returned from the United States to South Africa with such enthusiasm for working with infants and children with AIDS, was also faced with opposition from his own department of pediatrics. "So there was I, this so-called superspecialist, who had come from America and knows everything. I didn't even have a consulting room."

Even when they had departmental support, those who sought to create clinics could face impediments that at every turn made their efforts more difficult. Paul Kocheleff brought with him a vision of what a clinic should be from his earlier work in Burundi, a site providing nutritional and psychological support, as well as the management of opportunistic infections. Central to him was the creation of a clinical space where patients "had the possibility to talk and to be treated as human beings." But space was a problem. Jeanne Dixon, who worked with Kocheleff, struggled to find rooms where patients could be seen.

We had no venue for our HIV/AIDS clinic. When Paul arrived, I would check which clinic had finished and ask for permission to use the consulting room. We would move all our patients to the venue and start the clinic. On occasion, the medical or urology doctors would come back and we would have to find another venue. We could move venue three times during our clinic. Sometimes, we would find an empty room but the staff did not want us to use their venue because they didn't want it "contaminated." It sounds outrageous doesn't it? This was the mid-90s, and we struggled and we struggled, and management wasn't going to give us any help.

Even efforts to shift the burden of care for patients from hospital wards to community-based settings could encounter bureaucratic resistance. At the Church of Scotland Hospital, Tony Moll sought to develop an innovative home-based care program since the hospital, despite its complement of 350 beds, could not cope with the increasing numbers of patients. It was meant to be a part of his Philanjalo (Live Forever) Continuum of Care for AIDS, which already included hospital and hospice services.

In 1996–97, we were inundated with patients starting to come into the hospital with opportunistic infections. We were out there on our own in this rural hospital, and we would have to deal with what we had coming through our hospital gates. We realized then that this was going to be something really big. And when it hit us at Tugela Ferry, it would be universal across the province, and we would not be able to transfer our patients somewhere else.

It was in that environment that we came across the concept of home-based care and bringing on our community as partners to help us look after our terminally ill patients, to get them involved because we could see that our resources within the hospital were completely limited. We went to the matrons, and we said that we want to hold a home-based care training session. They said, "What's that? Where is the circular from the Department of Health saying that you must do that?" It took quite a long time to convince our matrons and the administration staff that this is a feasible response.

The End of Innocence

The resistance that clinicians confronted as they sought to face the emerging AIDS epidemic occurred in a context that at least superficially suggested that the national government and the Ministry of Health under the leadership of Nkosazana Zuma understood full well the need to forcefully address the threat. But there were early signs that the optimistic assumptions, following the election of Nelson Mandela in 1994, would not long persist. Disturbing tendencies in the ANC government soon began to affect AIDS policy. The first encounter, involving a play, *Sarafina II*, would suggest that the intimate consultative alliance forged between the government and the nongovernmental organizations that emerged in response to AIDS would be subject to deep strains. The second, involving the drug Virodene, was much more troubling, because it compelled scientists and physicians to acknowledge that the new national leadership would view with skepticism, if not hostility, critical debate about the direction of AIDS policy.

Concerned about the need to make a dramatic impact on the popular understanding of the threat posed by AIDS, Health Minister Zuma struck upon the idea of employing the skills of South African playwright Bongani Ngema to use theater as effectively as he had in his 1988 anti-apartheid musical, *Sarafina*. Quarraisha Abdool Karim, who had been appointed director of the AIDS office in the Ministry of Health, recalled that the goal was to do something "that goes on the road, gets to rural areas, gets to townships, the places where your electronic media and billboards don't get to." At initial meetings, the playwright suggested that a million rand would be required. In time, he tripled that figure. Then, to her dismay, Abdool Karim discovered that the final contract issued was for a startling 14 million rand. Delays followed, as the target dates for performance of *Sarafina II* came and passed. When she inquired regarding the status of the script, Abdool Karim was told by the playwright that he did not have scripts, that they would emerge in the process of performance. When she attended a rehearsal, she was "horrified" at what she saw. Eventually, the play appeared in May 1995, six months after the planned opening.

In early 1996, an investigative reporter began to track the story. Abdool Karim recalled, "I think it was the first real test the new government faced, and it turned out to be a real crisis, because they had no idea how to respond. What I thought was simple: be honest. 'We know we had made a mistake' was an unacceptable approach."

While some saw the entire story as a simple case of governmental ineptitude, others were more troubled. Clarence Mini remembered that, as a result of his public criticism as a leader within the National AIDS Convention of South Africa, Zuma was furious and did not speak to him for a year. For James McIntyre, who had served on the national coordinating committee of NACOSA, the events might have been viewed as a mere "hiccup," but the implications were far more distressing.

> I think that the *Sarafina* debate, the passions that were aroused, was kind of the end of the era of innocence. Everybody thought that everyone would work together. The government was going to carry on in this lovely consultative South African way and listen to everybody and do what they wanted. I think *Sarafina* blew that apart. Because what you saw was a government turning in on itself, defending itself, not open to criticism. The communication lines were completely broken down. Nobody was talking

to anybody. From that time on, there was a move by government to sideline NACOSA.

The bitter controversy over Virodene soon followed.[4] Upon finding that the chemical agent killed HIV in the laboratory, three University of Pretoria investigators, none with AIDS research experience, believed that this industrial solvent, used in freezing animal organs, could provide an effective treatment for AIDS. Gary Maartens, who had long been involved with AIDS research, recalled the sequence of events that brought the putative cure to national attention.

> So they went from that observation, which was barely an observation at all, to decide this would be a good treatment for HIV. They put it in a plaster patch to apply to the skin to treat HIV, without really doing any of the primary work that was required. They sought ethical permission from the university to do a study. The university said no. But they carried on anyway.

Made aware of the Pretoria researchers' findings, the minister of health was taken by the idea that South African scientists could have an achievement that had eluded those in the developed world. She brought the team to a cabinet meeting, where they were greeted enthusiastically, as they sought funds to extend their work. The Medicines Control Council, the official South African regulatory body, was asked to approve a formal clinical trial. Maartens, along with others, was requested by the council to review the evidence. "The data were laughable. The solvent is a known toxin to the liver. There were serious doubts about toxicity, and there was no convincing evidence of efficacy. The numbers were tiny. And it was unethical; it was a complete disaster."

On the basis of such evaluations, the proposed trial was turned down. And at that juncture, a political furor erupted. With the perspective of someone who soon thereafter would become involved in other battles with the government over AIDS treatment, James McIntyre recalled that Thabo Mbeki, then deputy president, "wrote to most of the major newspapers attacking the council for not believing that there could ever be an African cure, suggesting that everybody was in the pay of the pharmaceutical companies." These were themes that would reappear when, as president, Mbeki would become embroiled in a conflict over whether HIV was the cause of AIDS, which would pit him against South Africa's scientific and medical establishment. Furious at the roadblock that had been erected, the government placed enormous pressure on Peter Folb, the control council's head and a professor of pharmacology at the University of Cape Town. At one point, Health Minister Zuma chastised him, "You're ANC. Why won't you back me on this?"[5] "It was," said Maartens, "just unbelievable."

For Jerry Coovadia, who had been appointed by Abdool Karim to chair a national AIDS and STD advisory committee, "it was during that period that a gradual alienation of most of us from the government on its approach to AIDS began. It was Virodene one minute, it was *Sarafina II* next." But for Coovadia, the turn of events had even more disturbing implications about the ways in which respect among political comrades, forged during long years of struggle, no longer prevailed. "I did as much for the struggle as many of my colleagues. Why didn't they ask us? Did they think that, as an Indian, I was not trustworthy? What was it? I don't know. It was some paranoia or some arrogance, which had crept in."

3

The Burdens of AIDS

Treatment and Its Discontents

It was not simply indifference and hostility with which those committed to caring for people with HIV had to contend. They were, in addition, confronted with pervasive denial and fear on the part of their patients. Those who were sick often sought to mask the nature of their maladies from family, friends, and neighbors. Denial and fear were, in turn, embedded in a radical therapeutic impotence that informed the world of AIDS care in the epidemic's first decade in South Africa. This was the context within which nurses and doctors began to forge their efforts to care for people with HIV.

Discovering HIV

As they began to show up in clinics, hospital wards, and the offices of private practitioners, patients afflicted with diseases which suggested that they had AIDS were often pressed to undergo HIV testing so that more definitive diagnoses might be made. But what seemed to doctors so obviously the right thing to do often met with resistance. Many patients responded by asking, What was the point of it? What was to be gained? At King Edward VIII Hospital, Anisa Mosam, a dermatologist, was not uncommonly rebuffed by her patients.

> We deal with this daily in the clinic. I see a patient with herpes zoster infection, and at that time they've got nothing else wrong. And they are shocked when you ask them to get tested. I can put my head on the block and tell them they are probably positive, but they'll say "No, I am fine." They would say, "Why, what can be done?" Or the other response is, "I am afraid, no, no, no." They are too afraid to think about it, because it's been associated with death. It's very difficult for us to convince them to have the test.

For clinicians who believed that the HIV test was essential to the most basic care for patients whose symptoms suggested that they were infected, such refusals could be the source of great frustration. Ramesh Laloo Bhoola expressed his despair over such patients in his private practice in Durban.

> You're really helpless. I saw a person who died this week. I saw her a year ago. She wouldn't allow me to check her HIV status. She came in this time with dehydration. The family dumped her and went. She looked HIV positive. I treated her; she died the next day. Exactly why she died, I don't know. She was only 34.

Hannah Mothshedisi Sebitloane, a Black obstetrician who, like Anisa Mosam, worked at King Edward VIII, shared the skepticism of her patients about the value of HIV testing in the 1990s, soon after she had finished medical school.

> Sometimes patients didn't understand why you wanted to do the test. You would have to explain that it has implications for her health and for that of the baby. And we would have difficulty sometimes to say why are we particularly interested in her HIV status. One of the patients asked me, "How is it going to change my management?" And, quite frankly, she had a point, because we didn't have much to offer her apart from the routine we would do for whatever condition she would have. It would really not make a difference to what care she received.

But despite her ambivalence, Sebitloane believed that the test was useful to doctors, and perhaps to their patients, in the instance of obstetrical surgery.

> Sometimes, the results of the HIV test would be important for us. Sometimes, we had to know, so that we could at least be more careful and more cautious, especially when we ended up having to do a delivery or a cesarean section. Then it would be necessary for us and those women to know. Sometimes, we would find that maybe they had a complicated delivery. Then, sometimes, we would cover her with an antibiotic, just so that you could prevent complications.

The rejection of voluntary testing was intimately linked to the widespread pattern of denial and the devastating implications of knowing the truth. Eula Mothibi described the stark scenario of illness and death that was playing out in Cape Town when she arrived there in 1997 to work in a community health center. People lived in denial in order to hide their disease, while others scrutinized them in order to uncover their secret.

> I saw a lot of people, men, coming from Johannesburg and coming home to die. And a lot of them thin, emaciated, and no one had been tested for HIV.

There was just this secrecy, this denial, and people talked behind closed doors. "Oh, did you see that one? Looks like he's got it! She looks like she's got it."

In Pietermaritzburg, Neil McKerrow, head of the Pediatrics Department at Grey's and Northdale, the city's previously white and Indian public hospitals, respectively, was able to map a genealogy of patient denial and its relationship to testing.

In the early 90s, if we had a child who came into the hospital with what we thought were symptoms of HIV infection, we would sit down with the mother and say, "Mrs. Dlamini, you brought Sipho here with the following problems. We find the following things when we look at him. We are very worried about an underlying problem giving rise to all of these issues. We would like to exclude HIV, because if it is HIV, we can look at how we can help you, and if it isn't, we can start looking for another cause." In the early 90s, the reply would be, "That's a white problem, and I am Black." When we got to 1993–94, it would have been, "That's a rural problem, and I come from the city," or vice versa, "That's a city problem, and I come from the country." By 1996, they would say, "Yes, it's quite possible. Please test." By 1997–98, they didn't want to know. And the interesting thing is, in the 1997–98 era, the more educated the family, the more they didn't want to know about it. They said, "Yes, you can test if you want, but we do not want to know. We cannot deal with it, so don't tell us."

Patients might also reject testing for practical, economic reasons. Andrew Ross, who was then at the 250-bed Mosvold Hospital near the Mozambique border, recalled discussions in which patients asked, "What can you offer me? If you test my blood and I die, my family won't get the funeral payout that we've been paying for. HIV is an exclusion factor." Some doctors neither counseled nor asked permission to test, rejecting the emerging human rights–based standard of requiring informed consent. They found their justification in the need to provide the best treatment to patients who might refuse to have their blood screened for HIV. One doctor explained why she was still testing without patient consent as late as 1998:

You just have to do the most you can do in the prevailing circumstances. If you know you can treat the chronic diarrhea, if it's not due to anything else untreatable, then you treat that. You are treating the symptoms and not the patient really, because most of the time patients would refuse to be counseled; they would refuse to be tested. So you ended up testing the patient anyway, because you wanted to know if the patient had HIV or not.

Others tested patients simply so that they could make a diagnosis to their satisfaction. At one of AngloGold's health centers, an HIV specialist reported that, even in 2004, after patients refused to have their blood assayed, some doctors would substitute alternative tests to confirm the presence of immune suppression. They would test for CD4 levels, a mark of immune suppression, the normal range for adults being between 800 and 1500. According to Kathryn Mngadi:

> The sad thing is that if a patient refuses an HIV test, which they often do, there are one or two doctors who will do a CD4 count anyway and make a diagnosis of HIV based on the CD4 count. And the medical record card— it's almost like the game "telephone," where you whisper something in someone's ear and by the time it comes back to you, it's totally different. So someone will write "query HIV," and someone will put "HIV test refused," and then someone will do a CD4 count, and five pages from there the patient is HIV positive. Most of the time, the CD4 is not done to tailor the management or the investigation that they've done, but just to say, well, this person is indeed HIV positive. Mine doctors—and maybe I'm not being fair—my perception is that they're a very gung ho bunch of generalists.

Some Black doctors felt that colleagues might use HIV testing to confirm their own sense of moral superiority and to stigmatize those with the disease. Eula Mothibi was deeply suspicious of the motives of the white physicians with whom she had contact. As one of relatively few Black African doctors, she was painfully aware of the racial and class differences between senior staff and their patients.

> Because a lot of the physicians were white men looking after Black patients, there was already that wide gap. Now, you've got these Black people who are coming in with this disease, and they got it because of their immorality. It was mainly Black people, and not just Black people, but the out-of-society sort, the prostitutes, the mine workers, uneducated. What almost came through was, it's good that they've got it, good punishment for them, there's too many of them in this country anyway. Black men, die off. That's very harsh, but those were the kinds of undertones.

It was within that context that some began to believe that Blacks were at greater risk of being tested without their consent. According to Nontuthuzelo Ntwana, a nurse in her late 30s who was raised in the impoverished eastern Transkei, now the Eastern Cape Province:

> Some of the patients were not diagnosed with HIV, especially the whites and so-called Colored people, even if the signs and symptoms were

there. They always ask, "What is this for? What are you doing now?" So if you're African, a doctor can just come and take blood, no explanation, nothing.

The daughter of a teacher forced into political exile under apartheid, Ntwana responded by refusing to cooperate with the doctors, despite her status as a nurse.

When the results are back, they will call you as a nurse to come in and disclose now. So that's when I got cross or not to be liked by some of the sisters, because I was sometimes the only person that could speak, translate for the doctor. I always did not want to interpret for that, and they would say, "You are the only one." But I said, "Does this patient know what you did before? Now, I must just tell this patient that she is HIV positive, and you didn't tell her before what you are taking this blood for?" So I always refused to interpret for that, especially if the patient didn't know before-hand.

Elizabeth Fielder, who worked as a nurse with Frank Spracklen at Cape Town's Somerset Hospital, witnessed the shift of its AIDS population from white gay men to Colored and then Black men, women, and children. Surgeons at Somerset in the early 1990s commonly neither counseled their patients about testing nor sought their consent.

A lot of the doctors in the clinics didn't do pretest counseling. We know that pretest counseling is so important, because if you pretest counsel the patient sufficiently, then posttest counseling is quite easy. That's what people are scared of, giving people the results. If you speak to them properly at the beginning, it's not that difficult to tell them. But people didn't understand this.

She recalled one of many occasions when a patient, unaware of why he was there, had been unceremoniously referred to her service.

I remember having a call from a surgeon who had diagnosed a patient, had just done a test—no pretest counseling, nothing—just taken a blood test. He was HIV positive and, of course, there was great panic. Before I knew it, I had this patient sitting in front of me with a letter from the surgeon, "This patient is HIV positive." So I said to the patient, "Has the doctor let you know?" He hadn't even told him. In the end, we had to tell the patient.

To address the fears surrounding the HIV test and the pattern of often sur-reptitious screening without consent, doctors and nurses committed to the interests and rights of their patients made a special effort to develop the clinical skills necessary to protect those who might be subject to abuse. They not infrequently had to press their hospitals to develop formal policies prohibiting testing without consent.

At Johannesburg's Baragwanath Hospital, James McIntyre initiated a voluntary counseling and testing program following the accidental discovery of antibodies to HIV in a number of his obstetrics patients in 1987 by the South African Blood Transfusion Service. His commitment to the right of patients to refuse testing played out on a larger scale, as he confronted surgeons and other doctors who felt that HIV tests should be used by clinicians to protect themselves.

> There was a big debate around 1991 about the rights of health care workers. It was driven by people from this hospital who very firmly believed that HIV testing should be mandatory, that nobody should be seen in the surgical ward until they were tested, and that surgeons should have the right to refuse the operation. I was actually part of a panel with Edwin Cameron [the gay human rights lawyer] and others who were trying to draw up guidelines for informed consent and the role of testing within medical settings. In this hospital, once we started the HIV clinic, there was a much greater awareness of the rights of people with HIV.

Breaking the News

While some clinicians believed that voluntary testing made the disclosure of HIV infection less onerous, many found imparting such results extraordinarily wrenching under any circumstances. Pediatrician Leon Levin, in Johannesburg, was mindful of the implications of telling a mother that her child was infected: "It's not just a simple issue. Not only are you breaking news about the child, you're breaking news about the mother, and very often the father as well. You're wrecking the family by giving them the news." He went on to describe the emotional impact of such disclosures.

> You've got to be there to know what it's like. We've used the word "heartbreaking." Your heart just sinks, just sinks to get the diagnosis back. It hits you and then you have to break the news. It's hard. There's no question that it's hard. The devastation on people's faces, it's something you'll never get used to. As the treatment has progressed, it's very easy to color it and say, "Look, it's not as bad as it seems." But in the old days, when you had nothing, no treatment, it was just devastating news.

Saul Johnson, who, like Levin, was trained at Baragwanath in pediatrics, was similarly moved when he described how difficult it was to report the results of a positive HIV test.

It was horrible! It's a horrible, horrible experience. There's not really anything to soften the blow, and you have to be honest. Some of them—you could see—were turning out to be the more long-term, nonprogressor type of pediatric HIV, and those were difficult on the one hand because sometimes the mothers didn't suspect it, but at least you could also say, "Your child could still live a long time."

Finding the words to communicate with and console their patients as they delivered their bad news was not easy. Margaret Shangase, who had years of nursing experience before she encountered AIDS at Pietermaritzburg's Edendale Hospital, remembered her initial patient with HIV. The pain she endured when, for the first time, she informed someone of his seropositive status left a lasting memory.

He was a young male of 22 years. He presented with so many opportunistic diseases that eventually he had sores from head to toe. The doctor decided to take his blood for testing for HIV antibody, and the result came back positive. And I was called to come and do the posttest counseling on this gentleman. Well, when I broke the news, he just cried and cried, and I couldn't help it, I also ended up crying. I tried to hide myself, but I couldn't. So we would both cry. And at the end of it, when we stopped crying, I started counseling him. He was the first patient; he was so precious to us all.

Few had the skills required. Eula Mothibi recalled an experience in 1992, when she was a 27-year-old intern, that underscored for her how little doctors understood about counseling. It was from a nurse that she had had to learn.

Those days, for us, people knew very little about proper pretest counseling, so it was, "Mama? Can we take your blood for a test?" And the woman would say, "Yes, doctor." That was it. And when the test result comes back, the senior doctor would come and say, "The test is positive, so you have to talk to her." And there was a senior nurse who was working in the medical department—a very good woman—she taught me a lot about counseling, and she came and went to tell the lady that the test is positive. In her words, "It doesn't mean you're going to die now. You'll have a good life. It will be all right." That was posttest counseling then.

Hannah Mothshedisi Sebitloane was unusually candid as she described her own limitations. She remembered one patient at King Edward VIII, a pregnant woman whose two previous babies had died and who had just learned from Sebitloane that she was infected.

She broke down crying that particular day, and I just sat there. I didn't do much. Then I left her, and I came back again to find out what does she understand about being infected, about the implications to the baby. I decided to walk away because I didn't really know what more to say, and most of the time I find that I am at a loss for words. You say to people, "I understand." Sometimes, I feel I don't really understand.

Patient Denial

Given the climate surrounding AIDS, the intimations of promiscuity and early death, patients struggled, often desperately, to hold the news at bay. Kogie Naidoo described the shock with which mothers at King Edward VIII hospital reacted once they heard that their child was infected.

> Most of the time, it is denial. They ask you, "Is it possible that the baby was swapped in the nursery? Is it possible that my neighbor breastfed the child and infected the child in that way? Could the child have gotten the HIV by sitting in your queue, which is full of babies that are infected in this way?"

Unable to reconcile themselves to their diagnoses, perhaps too depressed to act, some patients sought resolution by shutting themselves off from whatever medicine could offer. Nontuthuzelo Ntwana, who worked at the MSF clinic in Khayelitsha, recalled a home visit that left her troubled.

> The patient was very sick, lying in bed. She was vomiting. When I got there, the treatment, the antibiotics, was still there; she didn't take anything. When I asked the patient, "Here's the tablets; can you not swallow it? Why are you not taking the treatment for opportunistic infection?" She couldn't answer. That was very bad. I came back to the clinic. The following week, we heard that the patient had passed away. If the person didn't accept the diagnosis, and if the person living with HIV doesn't want to live any longer, you can emphasize to do this and that, but he won't take anything.

English-born and -trained Ann Barnard came to Mosvold Hospital in rural KwaZulu-Natal in 1997 upon arriving in South Africa. She described a neighbor who "went downhill very quickly. He just wouldn't admit what was going on and wouldn't let us help him at all. He ran off to Durban, and we heard he was in hospital there, and he died down there eventually." Sister Margaret Shangase spoke of one of her former student nurses:

> I remember a nurse; she was doing a second year. She used to have perianal abscesses. The doctor decided to take her blood. It came back positive. When I broke the news—she was a very young girl, I think she was

17 years—oh, she cried and cried. And she said, "No, it's not true. This was my first boyfriend. It's not possible. You are telling a lie." She wouldn't just accept it. She didn't take long to die. She could not accept it.

Refusals to acknowledge an HIV diagnosis were not uncommonly suffused with deep shame. Helga Holst, the medical superintendent at McCord Hospital, described a young patient who took her own life after doctors revealed to her the results of her HIV test.

I was on call one weekend and asked to come urgently; someone had jumped out the window, a girl in the female medical ward who had been diagnosed with TB and was very, very wasted. At her bedside, I saw a Bible and something written inside it. She had been told that day she was HIV positive. The female medical ward is on the second floor of the hospital and the windows are quite high up. She must have been lying in her bed looking at the window. She got herself up, jumped onto her bedside table, and jumped out, because she could not face the condemnation that would come from her church and from her friends that she was HIV positive. So I found her lying at the bottom of this window on the concrete with her head twisted to the side; I think she had a broken neck, and she was dead. The security guards lifted her up and put her on the trolley, and we carried her into the hospital again.

The response of many poor women to their diagnoses was a reflection of the economic and social dependency that defined their relationships with men and of their need to protect their children. AIDS also raised the specter of violence. The prospect of informing their partners could be terrifying. In Johannesburg, Leon Levin noted that if the mother "told the father, or the father found out, he'd run away, or beat her up. That's changed a bit, but it hasn't changed much; they're still very judgmental, much in denial, and blame the women."

Caroline Armstrong, working in the AIDS clinic at Grey's Hospital, confirmed Levin's observation, while underscoring the inequalities that limited poor Black women's freedom of action.

It's really frustrating. You just say to the women, "I really think you should tell them." And the answer is usually one that I've got no defense against. They say things like, "But he'll kill me," and they don't mean it jokingly. Or "he'll beat me and leave me." What can you say? They must just keep quiet.

Kogie Naidoo, herself a mother, described the dilemma she experienced when she, as a pediatrician, had to inform a mother with meager resources and choices that her baby had AIDS.

She is unemployed, so she is afraid to confront the partner regarding her HIV status for fear of having the roof over her head and that of the child removed. She is economically dependent on him. She feels all this anger towards him, but she can't deal with it for fear that she is going to be thrown out. You are adding to her burden by giving her a diagnosis that her child has AIDS, and you can do absolutely nothing for her. In a sense, you had to tell her because she needed to be prepared in terms of her own emotional resources and how she is going to use them, repeatedly, in the hospital. She needs to be prepared because she has to allocate money for bus fare to come. So you are faced with a dilemma each and every time you are faced with giving a mother the news.

It was not only women who feared disclosure. The reasons that miners gave for not disclosing to their wives deeply resonated with the history and mores of the migratory labor system. These men led two lives, one in the overwhelmingly male world of work, single-sex hostels, liquor outlets, and prostitution, much like a military encampment, and the other in their rural villages, where their dependent families remained, historically barred from accompanying these workers by the mine authorities and later by the apartheid laws. HIV forced the men to find a way to bridge the two worlds. Kathryn Mngadi, head of the HIV wellness clinic in Orkney in 2004, described their dilemma:

I had a patient who said, "When I'm at the mine, it's like I'm a different person from when I'm at home. At home, I'm a father and husband. I only go home every six months, and by that time they've collected all the problems and issues of six months, and they wait for me to make these decisions. I come home with money, and I'm only there for a month. How do I tell my wife I'm positive and, a month later, leave? What does she do then? Who does she turn to? And if she leaves me in the meantime and leaves the children, what do I do? And then when I come to the mine, I'm here with a whole lot of women that are clamoring because they want money, and I'm so popular. It's like I'm two different people! I can't go home and tell my wife." I really feel his turmoil.

A Conspiracy of Silence?

Privacy and confidentiality were meant to protect patients against discrimination, embarrassment, or harm and to allow them some control over their lives. By acts of omission or commission, doctors and nurses sought to keep their patients' HIV diagnoses invisible to the prying eyes of relatives. At King Edward VIII, Sister Gabi Mbanjwa recalled:

We had a protocol not to write that the patient is HIV positive, because during visiting hours the relative usually comes. We hung the file against the foot of the bed. And on the sheet is written the patient's name, diagnosis, etc. The doctor only writes what the patient presents with. But the relatives, they go as far as paging through, wanting to know what is actually wrong with the patient.

As the number of infected patients increased, the staff at King Edward VIII developed codes to indicate HIV infection on their charts and records, but these were quickly noticed and cracked by the patients: "Sister, I've seen here the doctor wrote RVD [retroviral disease]. That means I'm HIV positive. And my parents are going to come."

There were doctors committed to the welfare of their patients who were sharply critical of the expectation that professionals maintain the strictest confidentiality. Tony Moll, whose extraordinary work would make the Church of Scotland Hospital a showcase of AIDS care in a rural setting, was critical of a confidentiality that, he felt, could serve as a gag rule. It prevented clinical colleagues from offering information or receiving advice and masked the growing force of the epidemic in the community.

It was a climate in which we as doctors were working in the 1995 to 1997–2000 period, where you would attend Department of Health meetings where they would say, "Confidentiality is absolutely essential." We all understand that, but it went to the extent that if I had an HIV patient and I took that patient to [the operating] theater, I was not allowed to tell the theater sister that this person was an HIV patient. So it wasn't even "shared confidentiality" that was allowed. Some hospitals had the problem where a nurse or the counselor would interview the patient, and the patient would test positive, and the doctor who is treating the patient would not be told that the patient was positive. We were not allowed to write "HIV," "immune compromised," or anything like that on death certificates. It was this absolute secrecy that was like a heavy dark blanket above our heads within the hospital, where we were restricted [in] talk[ing] to one another as colleagues even about our patients. You certainly couldn't talk to family members about the diagnosis, so that family members understood the cause of death as TB, pneumonia, chronic diarrhea. So nobody knew that people were dying of AIDS in our community.

But secrecy meant preserving a silence that could affect the welfare of others. As long as those who had tested positive refused to disclose their status to others, doctors and nurses became complicit in what Ann Barnard called "a complete conspiracy of silence." Eula Mothibi described a Cape Town patient whom she found to be personable and amusing, but who refused to accept his diagnosis, a predicament that she treated lightly but could have easily turned tragic.

> There was a man in our ward, Mr. Smith. I looked after him for a long time, and he had HIV and TB. He was married. He had a wife and two sons. Thank God, the wife was not infected. She was nice and plump. I would spend time with her. He denied totally that he had HIV/AIDS. He was so skeletal, so emaciated and wasted, and I got very close to him. Everyone knows he's got HIV/AIDS, and he's saying, "No, no, I don't have HIV. I just have TB. Doctor, tell them it's just TB." And then, we would release him home; he'd get sick, and he'd come back in again. But Smith's story was very sad, because he was giving his wife a hard time. Every time he went home, he would demand intercourse with the wife. She told me, "Look, we were using condoms, but now, doctor, I'm very scared, so I don't want to do it." So, I would be in the middle, saying, "Smith, look, you're a reasonable man. You've got two kids. We are very fortunate that your wife's not infected. Let her look after the kids." "But doctor, when I go home, I want to! What must I do?" Eventually, he passed away.

For Bongani Thembela, who had treated AIDS patients in a number of public hospitals in KwaZulu-Natal and had witnessed the consequences of nondisclosure within his own family, preserving patient confidentiality could be irresponsible and deadly. Speaking in 2004, he said:

> I used to believe that confidentiality was sacrosanct. But I now believe that confidentiality may be criminal, because people don't disclose, and the medical profession supports this. I have seen people from within my family where one was positive whereas the other one was negative. And, subsequently, the other became positive. Although I can never say 100 percent, it becomes obvious to me that the one has infected the other, when it could easily have been avoided by disclosure. And by the time they disclose, it's too late. They are on their deathbed. I really feel that as long as there is no malicious intent, confidentiality should be done away with. I've seen too many people die, who I feel could have been saved if we didn't have confidentiality.

And so Thembela came to believe that doctors had a duty to inform unsuspecting partners, a position long advocated by conservative critics of the preeminence afforded to privacy in shaping AIDS policy and practice in South Africa.

> I look at it as my job. If people are committed to each other, even if they are not married, I disclose now. I always tell. I say, "If you don't, I will." I always give them an opportunity to disclose. I have seen it happen in my

community, where disclosure has led to violence. That happens. But I still feel that, despite that, I am leaning more towards disclosure than not disclosing.

For others, the issue of disclosure went beyond the question of protecting the unsuspecting from HIV. To alert partners and family members, to encourage patients to disclose their infection would be to make public an epidemic which, because of stigma and confidentiality, remained shrouded in secrecy. Only in this way would the community be able to take full measure of the catastrophe before it. So felt Paul Nijs in 2004, two decades after he had emigrated to South Africa at the age of 36. Sitting in the Communicable Disease Clinic (CDC), the euphemistically named AIDS clinic at Edendale Hospital, he said:

On the issue of confidentiality, I was of the impression that by opening the doors, that eventually people will accept that this is a big problem and that you should be aware of it, that you should change your lifestyle because of it. To keep it fully confidential was to me to say it will never become a big issue. I was not really happy about the fact that we in the medical profession closed our eyes, that somebody could leave your consultation room and you knew that that person was HIV positive and that you didn't do anything about it.

I would have said, "Sit down, please. The chances are that you are HIV positive, that you have the disease are very, very high." I feel that it is my responsibility to do that. But you're not allowed to do that. You were supposed to say things like, "I suggest that you go to a counselor and that you are informed about HIV/AIDS." But it was all so vague, and there were in those days hardly any counselors. There was no structure, no people a patient could go to to explain, "This is HIV/AIDS; this is how it can affect you." It was kept all too confidential, and it had to stay confidential, because of the risk that they would be stigmatized, that they would be kicked out of the family. I'm not saying that there were no good reasons to think that confidentiality would be a good thing to do, but that confidentiality certainly had a very bad impact on the catastrophe. We are now 14 years into this epidemic and still it's an issue. In our ward rounds, I will ask the patient if he knows his HIV status; the nurse will actually lean over and whisper in his ear about a condition that is more common than common colds.

But, despite the fears of stigma and violence, despite the secretiveness that so many saw as a protective shield for the vulnerable and sick, patients did disclose, if often slowly and selectively. King Edward VIII's Sister Gabi Mbanjwa saw it as part of her job to encourage patients to share their diagnosis in order to gain support.

We didn't force the patient to tell their relatives, but during the counseling session, we tell them that it's nice to tell somebody in your family
what you are suffering from, so that they will be able to help you as time
goes on. We didn't force. But because we are doing ongoing counseling,
we just continue asking, "Are you not ready yet?"

For those who could not reveal their diagnosis to family, it was possible to find
succor with employers or friends. Sue Roberts, a nurse at Johannesburg's Helen
Joseph Hospital who came to AIDS work as a result of her interest in infectious disease,
described her attempts to help a young colleague disclose to someone she could trust.

I had a nurse who tested positive when she came [after] a needle stick
injury. She was very, very uptight and very emotional. It was very difficult
to handle for the first couple of days, and she actually said she wouldn't
tell anybody. We explored her relationships. And she had a friend, he's a
platonic friend; they actually share lodgings. I said, "Well, why don't
you tell him?" And she said no, she wouldn't, but three days later she came
back and she said she had told him. And she settled down incredibly just
by having told somebody.

Finally, for some, revealing their HIV status to their family or friends served
multiple purposes, as it does for those with other fatal diseases: outreach, con-
fession, reconciliation. Sue Roberts recalled one of the most moving experiences of
her professional life, when a 22-year-old woman could surmount her own anger
and depression to speak to those important to her about her illness. When Roberts
first met her in the hospital,

she had refused to be tested; she didn't want to be counseled. She had PCP,
and I said to her the chances that you are HIV positive are very high. And
she eventually decided she would be tested. She then said to me she
wanted to meet with her family. I organized a meeting. I told her I would
come in at visiting time when her family could all be there. I organized a
wheelchair for her and took her there. I was incredibly privileged to be
part of that meeting, because it was really to say goodbye to her family. We
had a prayer with the whole family. And then she went around to each
member of the family and friends who she had invited, and said thank you
for being there, thank you for doing this in my life; to the next one, we
were such friends in school and we remember these things that we shared.
Then she went on; to the one chappy, she said, "I was never really friends
with you because you were too close to my father, and I was angry at
my father because he made my mother work too hard. That's why we've
never been close; it's not because I don't like you." And then, eventually,
she said to them, "Now I must tell you that I have spoken to my doctors,

and they say that I've got AIDS and that I am dying." The next day, she died. I've often been with patients and their families, but to actually have somebody have the courage to be able to say goodbye in that way, I haven't come across before. She needed to get to that point, so that she could let go and die.

Creating Clinics

As was the case a decade earlier, when the first clinics were established for gay white men with AIDS, those who sought to meet the needs of poor Black women and men had to feel their way on terrain with few guideposts. As she and her colleagues at King Edward VIII were learning about AIDS, Raziya Bobat, who had seen her first child with AIDS in 1987, recalled that they had no medical treatment for infants or mothers, even against opportunistic infections. In its stead, she could provide only information.

> Basically, I would tell them that this is a new disease and that it is an infection and that it can pass from the mother to the baby or from the woman to her partner or vice versa. That was the extent of our knowledge. We didn't know that breastfeeding was going to cause a problem. The kind of thing we encouraged was immunization and good nutrition, and that was it.

Doctors in military hospitals could do little more for members of the South African Defense Force. A young doctor recalled with sorrow caring in 1995 for a colonel dying of AIDS, a patient with whom he had become particularly close over the long course of the illness. In describing the care he had provided to the officer, he remembered, "At that stage, we didn't do anything in the military, nothing; we tested for opportunistic infections, but no definite treatment." Although drugs were available in South Africa to treat tuberculosis and *Pneumocystis carinii* pneumonia, none were used in the instance of AIDS. "It was depressing, because we knew he wouldn't make it; and we knew we couldn't give him definite treatment. You don't give up, but you know you can't help him. It was depressing." Like others, his recourse was to offer counseling and other psychosocial services.

Clinical impotence was not limited to the public sector clinics and hospitals. Themba Mabaso, who opened his private practice in Durban in January 1993 when he was 30 years old, had diagnosed 20 HIV cases by the end of that year. Although a vigilant and careful diagnostician, he found his treatment options limited. "In 1992, there was nothing. In 1993, there was nothing I could do." Out of frustration, he turned to "psychotherapy," to counseling and hand holding.

> It was a question of explaining the disease process and what is likely to happen, explain the number of drugs that were on trial, and what a patient

needs to do between now and the time the drugs actually come, that they
may not work, that they may have side effects, there may be resistance.
It was just explaining exactly what I knew about the disease at the time and
just trying to give a positive outlook. At that stage, antiretrovirals like
AZT were still in the pipeline. We could treat opportunistic infections, yes,
but the treatment was always expensive.

Learning how to treat or care for AIDS patients resembled a voyage of discovery for doctors and nurses. In Durban, Henry Sunpath, 26 years old at the time,
began reading the AIDS literature in 1987. A few years later, Sister Gabi Mbanjwa
found some books for her purposes. Jeanne Dixon, a nurse who spearheaded the
AIDS program at Grey's Hospital, had a good librarian who sent her stacks of
journals. Lucky Ndokweni, in private practice in Durban, found workshops. In
those pre-Internet days, given the geographic and political distance between South
Africa and Europe or the United States, many doctors struggled to discover what
they needed to know. Often, they fell back upon trial and error, much as doctors
had in the United States in the 1980s. Not uncommon was the experience of
Mariëtte Botes, an Afrikaner doctor who has worked in both private and public
hospitals in Pretoria. The commencement of her AIDS education coincided with
her entry into HIV care, with admittedly mixed results. In 1994, the specialist in
internal medicine who had first organized the AIDS clinic in her hospital went
abroad, leaving a gap.

He was looking for somebody to take over his HIV clinic, although the
clinic saw only a very few patients at that stage. I was the only one willing to
take it over, not because I liked HIV, just because I was willing to do the
extra work. I knew nothing about HIV, absolutely nothing. Well, I like
communicating with patients, and I like to treat the small problems
that they have, and I started to learn all about it, and I read articles. So
I basically went on with the clinic, and I taught myself. There was nobody to
teach me. I think I made a lot of mistakes along the way. There was nobody to ask. We didn't have any contacts in Europe or the U.S. You just
accepted it. It was either me or another doctor, who knew less than I.

Eula Mothibi was luckier. Unlike many others who found themselves confronting AIDS, she was able to learn from experienced doctors, including Cape
Town's Gary Maartens, of whom she said, "He was so good. I got involved with
him and learned a lot from him; I just hung on to him. And over four years, I've
learnt a lot from him and taught myself—because there wasn't any education. No
one was interested in HIV/AIDS."

Learning occurred as efforts were made to extend clinical services. In the
early 1990s, James McIntyre created a clinic for pregnant women at Baragwanath
Hospital. In the process, he discovered that his careful efforts to eliminate

those physical barriers that might reinforce the HIV stigma–associated secrecy were viewed by his patients as an impediment to their own needs for mutual support.

> We decided to form a kind of specialized antenatal clinic for those women. We didn't have anything to offer them really, other than counseling and testing and support, and we took an approach that was trying to be holistic, that was trying to combine medical and psychosocial care. We started in what was a storeroom of the antenatal clinic here that we cleared out and opened up. We had four patients once a week and then five and then six, and it grew on from there. And from that process has developed the things that we've done since.
>
> Right at one end of the clinic, there was a wooden screen that divided the general waiting area. Every week, when we went down, I would move this wooden screen so that the waiting bench for our clinic was together with all the other mothers, so that they didn't feel that they were being blocked off. And every week, by the middle of the morning, the screen was back in place. We said, "Why?" And they said, "Because we like it here. We can talk to each other, because we know why we are here, why we are sitting here. So we can be open about what's happening."

The very effort to offer something different to the women who came to the clinic transformed the nature of the relationship he had with them. Inevitably, emotional bonds formed, unusual in the impersonal environment of public hospitals. While they enriched his work, they took a toll.

> What was unusual was that I was building up a one-on-one relationship with women in this hospital, much more like a private practice. Generally, we do 50 deliveries a day here, and a pregnant woman is lucky if she sees the same doctor twice in her pregnancy, never mind during her labor. What was happening within this clinic in the beginning and as it grew was that the doctors and nurses—it was really me and maybe a couple of other doctors who moved in and out and then Glenda Gray—we were forming very close relationships with women and having now to live through the death of their babies. Having to live with the fact that they had no job, that they had no support, that they were getting ill, that somebody was dying, that they got beaten up and thrown out of the house.

As other clinics were established, they too were compelled to go beyond the conventional medical models of care. With significant limits on what could be offered, they often focused on their patients' social needs. At Johannesburg Hospital, Leon Levin recalled with enthusiasm his creation of an HIV pediatric clinic in 1996.

I started seeing patients in the wards who needed long-term follow-up and yet weren't being followed up. The attitude in the hospital was that this is such a common disease that everybody should be handling it. And it worried me because you didn't have that happening with kidney diseases; you didn't have that happening with oncology. You had people who were specializing in the disease and giving the best possible care. And here what was happening was, yes, everybody was getting involved, but nobody was getting involved properly. And so I decided, this is not the way. We needed to formalize it, get a clinic going. The head of pediatrics, he was very supportive; he is a wonderful man. He supported me right through.

There wasn't much at that stage. What we were offering was prophylaxis against tuberculosis and PCP. We were following up with the children whose moms were positive. I was the only full-time pediatrician there. We had a social worker involved; we had a dietician involved in the clinic. So we chose Thursday afternoon because it was an open time, but also there was nobody else there. I didn't want the stigma of "Oh, it's the HIV clinic."

It was wonderful because it was just us. It was just the kids there and the moms with the young babies. You could see all the children running around. The amount of counseling that went on at the clinic just between moms giving each other support, because they all knew they were there with the same disease. And it was absolutely wonderful just to watch this and to see the older kids at school. And all the comfort that the parents took from seeing these older kids, knowing that it's not as bleak as they were led to believe. It was really a wonderful set-up. The nursing sisters who were involved brought other pulmonology sisters along. They were unbelievable. They had enough work to do, they didn't need another clinic, and yet they did it.

One of the most remarkable efforts took place at McCord Hospital in Durban. While the vast King Edward VIII Hospital did not create an adult HIV clinic until 2000, McCord had, in 1995, put together an outpatient clinical service designed to meet the medical, economic, psychological, and spiritual needs of its patients. Its first director, a Christian doctor, pressed the need for a clinic on a receptive and supportive administration headed by Helga Holst.

We'd see quite a lot of people coming in who were terminally ill with AIDS. They would be saying, "We've been to this hospital and we've been to that hospital," and they would list all the hospitals they'd been to and clinics, and everybody said, "There's nothing we can do." Being a Christian, I was looking for answers in the Bible. And the thing that struck me was the similarity between AIDS and leprosy in the Bible, how they would be rejected by their family, the same way lepers were just cast out and made to live apart from the community and had to ring a bell if they came near people. And I then looked at Jesus and his response, and he did an amazing thing in his time. He actually reached out and touched the leper. I began to realize that this, as a Christian hospital, me as a Christian doctor, we should be following Jesus's example. And even if we can't cure these people, there would be a lot we could do to help them and support them and their families. And so I spoke to our counselor, and we got together and decided to set up a clinic, which at that time just ran on a weekly basis.

The center is called Sinikithemba, which means "we bring hope." And the hope is really the hope of Christ and of eternal life. We believe it is important to die having committed your life to Christ. They know that they are going to an eternity with him, so it's not an end. And for me, that's what makes doing it all worthwhile.

Because the patients were very poor, and because the hospital, a state-subsidized but private institution, charged fees for its services, Sinikithemba confronted the need to help those it served to earn money. Thus began one of the clinic's most striking features. Henry Sunpath, who would become the director of the hospital's AIDS service, remembered how poverty provided the motivating force for this innovation.

People could not afford even basic medical care. It means they were the poorest of the poor. Patients used to often come to this place, just saying, "I'm very sick. I've got no money." The clinic began looking at creative ways to meet that need. The income generation project was one of those which involved beadwork and manufacturing of clothes. And out of this grew a core support group who formed a choir to sing hymns in Zulu and English. The Sinikithemba choir became the face of HIV to the world.

Although doctors and nurses in the public sector were already aware of the deep poverty endured by many of their patients, the early years of the AIDS epidemic provided them with dramatic experiences of how their patients lived. A world beyond the confines of clinical medicine was opened, exposing needs for food and shelter. For Tony Moll in Tugela Ferry, it was the home-based care that he had pressed to create that provided the opportunity to see his patients in a new way.

What the home-based care program did for me was that it took me out of the hospital, away from files, away from bedsides. I would visit patients sick in their own homes, and I would be on their own bed, sitting in their own lounge, seeing their own little children come in, seeing granny around. And somehow this brought a different dimension to it, because you became part of the family. You saw the person, not a diagnosis. This was now a living person with feelings, with a family, a disease that touched children who were going to become orphans, a disease which touched the family because now there was no longer an income.

Moll went on to recall his experience with one patient.

A woman in our tuberculosis ward developed a spinal complication and became a paraplegic. So we kept her in the ward. She was about 35. One of the sisters of the home-based care program brought to me a small scrap of paper that had been torn out of a school exercise book and on the paper was written in a very childish, Zulu handwriting, "Mummy please come home." The sister said, "Well, it's the eight-year-old daughter of this paraplegic patient, and she is saying 'Mummy, please . . .'" So I said, "Well, I think she stayed a month and let's take her home."

We packed her up in a van with her medications, with some food, and we took this lady home. We were met by her little daughter in a tiny hut that could barely house a single bed. It was an early winter morning. When I walked into the hut, I can remember just feeling the goose bumps on my arms and feeling that this is really cold. I looked up at the roof, and I could see that a lot of the thatch was missing; I could see the sky through the roof. This little eight-year-old had been living alone in this hut whilst her mum was in hospital, and she was fed by neighbors who just gave her what was left over. She was living on her own until she basically couldn't take it any more.

We saw that there was a huge social need there, and we managed to get the local church to fix the roof. We got a wheelchair for the mum. We got the little girl back to school. We made sure that there was an adequate supply of nutrition to the home, and we regularly visited this mother and her daughter. We walked a long path with this patient over a period of perhaps two years until she really wasted. We brought her into the hospice. It was as if she was almost a family member.

Sister Margaret Shangase's efforts at outreach in Pietermaritzburg provided her with a similar experience. Her reaction was all the more striking since, as a Black woman, the social gulf that could, in part, explain Tony Moll's response was not a factor. Two cases remained vivid to her despite the passage of time.

Sometimes, you have to park your car and walk about five kilometers before you reach the house. And what was worse, sometimes when I arrived at the place, you find a person lying in bed all by himself or herself.

I remember one day I knocked and knocked at the door. Nobody opened, until I asked the neighbor where were the people for this family. She said, "Inside, push hard." I pushed the door hard, and I found him. He was sitting with his head bent. I shook him up. I said, "I've been knocking for such a long time. Why don't you open?" He said, "I heard the knock, but I did not have the strength to go and open the door." I said, "What is it that is stopping you? What's happening to you?" He said, "Number one, I'm hungry. I last had food yesterday at lunchtime. I'm so weak that I cannot move." Secondly, his feet were so swollen. He said he couldn't put them on the floor, he can't balance, and they were painful.

Shangase went on to recall an equally poignant memory.

I was making a follow-up for a young woman. When I approached the door, I heard a cry inside. It was a two-year-old child, her daughter. She was crying bitterly. I asked her, "What's wrong with the baby?" She said, "She's hungry." I said, "Why don't you feed her?" She said, "I have nothing to feed her now." I said, "Why don't you breastfeed her?" She just undressed and showed me. Both breasts were just raw with sores. She said, "I cannot feed her." And she went outside. She didn't tell me where she was going; she just left me in the house. She went out and came back with an old electric iron. She said, "Please buy this iron so that I can get something to buy a bottle of milk." I bought the iron. I knew I was not going to use it. I gave her some money, and on the way back I had to throw it out.

Language

However committed were the clinicians who began to provide AIDS care, the context in which they practiced was strained by cultural and class fissures. Among the most striking, because it directly affected communication between doctors and those for whom they cared, was linguistics. White and Indian clinicians spoke Afrikaans or English or both. Few had a command of any of the languages of South Africa's Black population, despite the fact that nine of them—Sepedi, Sesotho, Setswana, siSwati, Tshivenda, Xitsonga, isiNdebele, isiXhosa, and isiZulu—were officially recognized in the new constitution. And while there were many Black Africans who spoke English and Afrikaans, that was far less true for those living in rural areas or those who had recently migrated to cities. The result, one doctor said, was that he could touch, prod, observe, and listen but not talk to his patients. For him, regrettably, caring for patients and trying to determine their symptoms too often took on the qualities of "veterinary medicine."

Henry Sunpath, who spoke Zulu, in part because his parents spoke Zulu despite being Indian, said of the situation:

> Considering our historical background in South Africa, many Zulu-
> speaking people come into the hospital expecting not to be understood
> and quite willing to use an interpreter. That is the accepted norm in any
> place that you go. And they do know that here are these people who really
> want to help us but they can't understand us, and we must help them
> understand us.

It would be too easy to understand the linguistic gulf simply as an expression of cultural or racial disdain. Martha Bedelu, a 29-year-old Ethiopian doctor who had come to South Africa to work with Médecins sans Frontières in its AIDS clinic in Khayelitsha, understood that her commitment to international humanitarian medical work would take her to many places where she could not speak directly to her patients. She did her best with interpreters, providing care that might not otherwise have been available.

> I usually use translators. To understand their pure medical problem is
> not difficult. It's not easy, it's not easy working with translators, but still
> I don't think it's very bad. One is always supposed to develop a relation-
> ship with patients; you smile with them, joke sometimes, and they feel very
> comfortable with you. And if you see them regularly, even if you don't
> speak the language of the patient you are treating, you definitely have a
> relationship with them.

Unlike Bedelu, Haroon Saloojee was born in South Africa. Despite his Indian background, he had chosen for political reasons during the apartheid years to define himself as "Black." But other than a few words, he could speak no African language.

> What we ended up doing was learning key words and doing this kind of
> stymied conversation where you threw out phrases like "Was the child
> vomiting?" or "Did the child have diarrhea?" or "Is the child crying?" You
> knew these key terms, and you could communicate at a very basic level.
> If that didn't work, then I would usually use an interpreter.

He understood the limitations this imposed on clinical communication, but had not found the time to change the situation.

As he assiduously worked to establish AIDS clinics in Pietermaritzburg, Paul Kocheleff, who had left his native Belgium two decades earlier to work in Burundi, was immediately struck by the linguistic barriers and their clinical implications.

Very few of the doctors can speak Zulu. The number of doctors in South Africa has decreased, and the South African doctors who probably couldn't speak Zulu have been replaced by doctors coming from different areas of the world. There were Polish, Bulgarian, some Belgian doctors, some from Burma, from India, from Pakistan. It's evident none of these doctors could speak Zulu. And unfortunately Zulu is a difficult language, and so the enthusiasm of the people to try to learn Zulu was very small. I didn't try to learn the Zulu language. So we had to use the help of translators. If you speak the language of the patient, to have a good history takes time. If you use somebody else to translate, it takes more time. And because of the number of patients, because of the lack of time, the quality of many histories was often poor.

Paul Nijs, a Belgian compatriot and coworker of Kocheleff, knew all too well the gulf created by his inability to communicate fluently with his patients, despite his efforts to speak basic medical Zulu.

I can now do a simple conversation. I would be able to find out what the problem is. When a patient explains, I will always listen. And I understand a lot, but I cannot really speak it. I'm also a bit afraid to speak the language, because they might laugh. It's difficult. A lot of patients have psychological problems, but we never touch them because of the language barrier.

Laura Campbell, who came to South Africa from Northern Ireland in 1991 and worked in Port Shepstone, south of Durban, underscored how utterly inadequate it was for her to rely on translators, especially given her concern about easing the suffering of her patients.

You ask the patient something like, "How are you feeling?" And then the patient gives a long, long, long answer, and the interpreter says that he is feeling fine. I say, "No, he didn't say fine; he said something more than fine." Especially when the patient is confused, the patient talks, talks, talks, talks. You ask, "What did he say?" and she would say, "He is confused, doctor," because they did a bit of psychiatry. You are trying to pick up subtleties, and you say, "But tell me exactly what he said." "He is just too confused, doctor." I have these few white patients and 99 percent Black patients, but once you chat to the white patients, you just realize what you are missing out on. So I think my philosophy is that it's always better than nothing, but it's virtually impossible to practice medicine as I would like to practice it.

James Muller, who bore major administrative responsibilities for the Department of Medicine in Pietermaritzburg's hospitals, had practiced medicine in

Canada in the late 1970s and so knew what it was like to be a clinician in a setting where resources were ample and language posed no obstacle to care. The terms he used to characterize his current work stressed briskness and efficiency rather than engagement.

> I can't communicate directly with many of the patients because I don't speak enough Zulu, and they don't speak enough English. It becomes a matter of assessing the clinical situation, making a working diagnosis, recommending appropriate therapy, and moving on to the next patient.

Remarkably, some have made peace with the barrier of language, despite their evident commitment to providing the best care possible for their patients. Tony Moll noted that, despite having been at the Church of Scotland Hospital for 17 years, he was still dependent on translators.

> It's not a barrier; it's something that one gets used to very quickly. In fact, because there are so many cultural issues that come out in a medical examination and explanation of signs and symptoms, it's good to have a Zulu person. It's usually a nursing sister that helps us along, because in the Zulu culture, our patients don't think in terms of infection and natural causes of the disease. Our patients are rural Zulu people. Their signs and symptoms are linked to their religion, and so their explanations of signs and symptoms can be very complicated. For instance, if you are asking, "Tell me about your abdominal pain," they could say, "My auntie did this," or "I stepped over a spell that was cast in front of me, and that's the origin of my disease." I would have to wake up as a Zulu person, and I think that would make a difference. I think there will always be the barrier of being a white person brought up in another culture.

Others who acknowledged the impossibility of traversing the linguistic divide sought out a patient population with whom communication was possible. This was crucial to David Spencer, who left the public sector for private practice in 2000. His work with gay men at Johannesburg Hospital had first brought him into contact with AIDS among English- or Afrikaans-speaking whites. For Spencer, a deeply religious man, speaking to his patients about their spiritual concerns and ministering to those needs was a defining feature of his practice. As AIDS become a disease of heterosexual Black men and women, he found that within the public medical services:

> You would be primarily English- or maybe Afrikaans-speaking; your patient would be Zulu- or Xhosa-speaking. You needed to communicate, particularly on death and these sorts of things. So the families would take

over and take the patient home, and there would always be a distance.
Much less now that I am in private practice. One of the joys I have in the
kind of work I do now is that my patients are more sophisticated, have
been educated, trained. They speak English. Where they're dying or where
you need to speak very deeply, they can understand it.

For those relatively few who made the commitment to learning an African
language—who saw the justifications "I am not a linguist" or "Zulu is simply too
difficult" as unacceptable—the task could be demanding. But in the end, they had
opened to them a level of communication that often transformed their understanding of their patients. Bernhard Gaede, who worked in rural areas and for
whom the immediacy of patient contact was a crucial part of the clinical experience, found that learning Zulu was transformative.

I wanted to speak Zulu because I wanted to know what is being said and not
what somebody thinks is being said. Once I started to understand Zulu,
I realized that there's just mountains that gets lost in translation. It's one
of these things that prevents me from blunting. It helps me to engage with
the person. It tells me so much more about what's actually going on.
I find it difficult to think about what it was like when I needed to use a
translator.

But having learned one African language did not resolve the problem of caring for
patients who spoke others. The contrast with his work in Zulu made it all the more
clear to Gaede how crucial it was to be able to listen unimpeded, to speak directly.
"When a person speaks Sotho or Venda, I find it difficult to work, because I cannot
concentrate on the patient. I don't understand what is being said; what the nurse is
telling me is not enough."

For Black doctors and nurses, there was an almost universal feeling that the
failure of white and Indian doctors to speak African languages represented a barrier
to the kind of care that could be provided by even the most devoted physicians.
Sister Gabi Mbanjwa recounted how the inability of doctors to understand Zulu
made intimate communication virtually impossible.

They tell us in Zulu, "Now you tell the doctor that I would like to speak to
[him]." You leave the doctor with the patient, but the doctor will call
you, "Sister, I don't understand what the patient says." The patient initially
does not want you to be there, but now, because the doctor is unable,
because of the language, you will be forced to be there. The patient will say,
"OK, it's fine," but it's not 100 percent OK.

Referring to non-Zulu-speaking doctors at Edendale Hospital, Sister Margaret
Shangase said:

Yes, they were missing a lot, a lot. Sometimes, the doctor would say something, and the patient answers something different from what the doctor is asking. Sometimes, the patient would tell the doctor, "I have a pain, a bending pain that starts from the foot, it goes up the calf, and it moves up to the hip," and you can see that the doctor doesn't understand what they are talking about in Zulu. And when he writes the history down, you can see. Sometimes, he writes one or two words, and you can see that he has missed the rest of the diagnosis.

Bongani Thembela, who worked for nine months with Paul Kocheleff and was acutely aware of the limits imposed by language at Edendale Hospital, ultimately left because of his dissatisfaction with what he could do at the clinic. At the end, he explained to his colleague how the gulf of race and language had affected patient care.

One of the reasons I find it painful to work in the clinic is that I think sometimes patients tell me things that they don't tell you, not because they don't want to tell you, but because they don't know how to tell you. I know what it is like to live in the township. I lived in the township.

What set many Black doctors apart from their white and Indian colleagues, even those who recognized the problem, was their vantage on what they understood to be the deeper issues involved. In South Africa, language is a matter with a long historical resonance. In the nineteenth century, Afrikaner intellectuals formally erected Afrikaans as a bulwark of ethnic nationalism against the ascendant English imperial ideology.[1] The Soweto uprising of 1976 was sparked by the apartheid government's effort to impose Afrikaans, which most Black Africans did not speak, as the official "medium of instruction" in Black schools. Veliswa Labatala, a nurse in Khayelitsha, characterized the linguistic barriers in South Africa as one of the scars left by apartheid ignorance. "Wherever you go here, you can speak English and Spanish, but if you speak Xhosa, you're insulting whoever you're speaking to. It's all political."

Lucky Ndokweni, today a doctor in private practice, had gone to study medicine in India, sent there by the African National Congress in the 1980s because his life was in danger. He had learned Hindi, but many of his patients spoke Tamil. As a foreign student, he was entitled to the assistance of an interpreter. He told his supervisor, "Madam, I applied for an interpreter, because I thought I would have a case that might speak quite deep Tamil." She said, "No, that's not right. Go and learn to speak Tamil. After that, you come back and sit for your final exam." And to his white and Indian colleagues who acknowledged their difficulties with language, he replied, "You guys were born here, you were born and bred in South Africa. I went to study ten years, ten years. I can speak two of the most important languages of India. I had to speak!"

In Cape Town, Eula Mothibi, like Labatala, saw the situation as the legacy of apartheid. About those who said it was simply too difficult to learn an African language, she said:

> It's difficult, but if your life depended on it, if you were told that you're not
> going to get a salary next month, you would learn it. It's just a matter
> of power. They feel more empowered. They feel they couldn't be bothered
> to learn the language. In this country anyway, the previously advantaged
> groups just want to carry that advantage and carry that power.

And from that perspective, complying with the request to translate for white or Indian doctors was tantamount to collaborating with an attitude Mothibi abhorred.

> When I was in school, even my student colleagues would say, "Eula, please
> ask him this." In those days, without thinking, I would ask the question.
> Coming here to Cape Town, I was a doctor in my own right, studying to
> become a physician. The professors in charge would be saying, "Eula,
> why don't you ask him such and such and such?" The defense I often used
> was, "Because I'm a Sotho, I don't speak Xhosa." And some of them
> know I speak Xhosa, so they would just look at me and grit their teeth and
> leave it alone. Sometimes, if it meant a lot for the patient, I would ask. It's
> a difficult situation, because in one way it might benefit the patient for
> them to get the information, and at the same time it just makes you an-
> gry. These people are treating this patient. They're supposed to be the
> patient's doctor, the patient's advocate. But if they can't speak to the pa-
> tient, how are they going to be the patient's advocate? How are they going
> to do what's in the best interest of the patient?

Traditional Healers

Language, however, was not the only broad cultural divide that separated most South African doctors from their patients. An equally important gulf existed in their understanding of disease, curing, and healing. And here the racial cleavages that had separated white and Indian from Black doctors in matters of language all but vanished. Doctors trained in medical schools, whether Black, white, or Indian, shared a scientific and professional world view that was utterly at odds with the cultural definitions of sickness and health still subscribed to by many of the Black men, women, and children whom they treated.

As they began to experience the symptoms of HIV disease, Black South Africans turned to traditional healers, who constituted a parallel health system existing in an uneasy relationship with allopathic medicine. When ill, those who needed care would consult sangomas, who divine the cause of illnesses and subsequently mediate with the ancestral spirits, and inyangas, who provided preparations, traditionally of herbal and animal origins, and rituals or symbolic offerings.[2] The South African Medical Association estimates that 80 percent of all patients employ traditional healers before turning to hospitals and clinics.[3] Many continue to use both systems of care simultaneously. But however they make use of traditional medicine, they then face doctors who, whatever their attitudes, almost never have contact with such healers.

James Muller was unusual in this regard, acknowledging relationships with traditional healers outside the hospital system in Pietermaritzburg, for which he has considerable administrative responsibility. He underscored the necessity of resisting the temptation to dismiss alternatives to conventional medicine as inherently inferior, and not simply for the strategic reasons more typically given by other doctors.

> It is quite often obvious that the patient has been to see a traditional healer because they have scarification marks on their skin. They are not reluctant to tell you. It's important not to be judgmental about it. Some people have the impression that traditional healers only do harm to their patients. My impression of traditional healers, in regard to first aid, is by and large they do good. There are instances where they do harm.
>
> I have some very good friends amongst traditional healers. I have been involved in negotiations with traditional healers about how they might be incorporated, and cooperate more closely, in providing appropriate health services to clients, and also to try and build systems whereby there can be mutual referrals between the two systems.

It was in dealing with tuberculosis—so commonly associated with AIDS—that Andrew Ross, who had been a principal medical officer and then the superintendent at Mosvold Hospital, came to appreciate fully why it was that his patients had first turned to traditional healers.

> Almost everyone in Ingwavuma in KwaZulu-Natal will visit a traditional healer before they come to see us at the hospital and probably after they have seen us at the hospital. If they have got TB and they are coughing or vomiting blood, they think that they have been bewitched. And if you've been bewitched, then you need to go and see a traditional healer, who needs to unbewitch you. It's no good going to see the white doctor; he knows nothing about bewitching. So, I wouldn't be the obvious first choice. And you need to believe that the bewitching has been dealt with before you take the TB medicines. Some of the traditional healers don't encourage people to take both their medication and Western medicines.
>
> When people have decided to come to us for treatment, we really try and encourage them to take our medicines. I think you really have to come from

a patient's world view. It's arrogant to feel that we are the authority on people's health conditions. If people feel that the traditional healers are making a contribution and that's their belief structure, I really believe that we have to respect that. If someone had meningitis and we really thought that we could treat it, and the family wanted to take the patient to see a traditional healer, then obviously we would try and negotiate that they stayed for ten days of treatment before they took them. But for children who appear to have AIDS, for whom we are not able to offer very much, then we have to be tolerant and say, "Well, this is part of your belief." It's very arrogant for us to be saying, "You can't take that child."

Having established some contact with such healers, Ross recognized that they could be useful in the emerging struggle against AIDS. He would say to them, "Can you be involved? These are the things that we think that you can do, and these are the things that we think you shouldn't be doing. In particular, you shouldn't be sharing blades when you make your scarifications."

For Bernhard Gaede, who began to work at Emmaus Hospital in rural KwaZulu-Natal in 2000, it was a commitment to holistic medicine, to viewing the process of healing as more than a mechanistic approach to symptom relief and cures, that made traditional medicine both interesting and valuable. It also made him skeptical of the oft-repeated stories about doctors and nurses being called upon to provide remedies for the damages suffered by those who had been ministered to by traditional healers.

We don't see the allergic reactions that we cause, that they see. So, I think we are doing as much iatrogenic damage as they do. Traditional medicine has been around for many, many generations and nations have lived with it, so it can't be that damaging. I also look quite a lot at traditional medicine approaches to integrating the different dimensions of the person into a healing process. Here, traditional medicine is streets ahead of us. We haven't got a clue of how to make a coherent meaning of HIV disease, so that the person can let go of it.

Drawing on his years of experience with medicine in Burundi, and acutely aware of how language was an impediment to coming to grips with the suffering of his patients, Paul Kocheleff was especially appreciative of what traditional healers could offer to his patients in terms of psychological support. "It took a bit of time to appreciate really, especially in the field of psychiatry, where they were fantastically useful. They deal with aspects of psychiatry much better than we could."

Such sympathetic perspectives were not only unusual but, when acted upon, generated institutional hostility that made the integration of the two very different systems of treatment almost impossible. Neil McKerrow, chief of pediatrics at Grey's and Northdale hospitals, recalled his frustrated efforts.

For us to get traditional healers into the hospital was totally impossible. I once managed to find one who was prepared to come to the hospital, and hospital management said, "What do you think you are doing, inviting one of those people into my hospital?" So, it was a no-no.

Acknowledging the deep cultural hold of traditional medicine, some thought it crucial to embrace a formally syncretic approach in an effort not to alienate patients. Sister Gabi Mbanjwa, head nurse at the HIV clinic of King Edward VIII Hospital, gave voice to the exquisite balance that had to be struck.

I do not say, "You must not." The patients need psychosocial support. So, now, if they tell you, "You know, Sister, I've been to the traditional healer," I say, "Good, but we have to do it in both ways because you are here now." But you don't crush them and say, "You shouldn't have gone. It's nice if you've been, it's fine, but now you are here. We're going to treat you, because you are suffering from this."

More common among caregivers in hospitals and clinics was an attitude of uncertainty, suspicion, and concern about how traditional approaches could interfere with whatever medicine had to offer. What especially troubled doctors was the way in which their medications could cause adverse reactions when mixed with the remedies provided by traditional healers. At a time when Western medicine had a limited range of effective responses to AIDS, this could be especially difficult. Pinky Ngcakani, who said that it was important not to be "too harsh or autocratic," urged her private practice patients in Durban to heed her warnings, though she knew that her appeals would often fall on deaf ears.

I'm sorry, I'm not trained to diagnose spiritual sicknesses. But when we come to a diagnosis, this is how I know to treat best. This is how I handle it really, because I don't know how else to. I know that there are medications available from traditional healers; but I can never vouch for them, because I don't know exactly how they work, what their side effects' profile is, and all sorts of things. But I wish that we could try this medication first, see how it goes. And people must not mix medication. Let's try and use this, give it a chance; and then if you feel this is not helping, then you can go on, instead of mixing everything. I know patients. They always try everything out of desperation.

Working alongside Tony Moll at the Church of Scotland Hospital in Tugela Ferry, François Eksteen was particularly concerned about how traditional medicines could harm young children. And unlike those who thought that the conceptual divide that separated doctors like him from traditional healers could be fruitfully overcome, he focused on the significance of the gulf.

Often the inyanga would administer the herbal medication as an enema.
They use a little hornlike instrument and actually insert it as an enema in
the child, or they can give it orally. Some of these oral medications are
quite innocuous, but others can actually be quite dangerous and precipi-
tate acute juvenile necrosis or acute renal failure in a small child or in a
baby that has already been severely ill from other causes. That's one of the
sad things that we regularly have to deal with, intoxications due to certain herbal medications.

They would say that their authority for using the medication is from
spiritual causes. But for me, it's not right from a scientific, empirical,
observational basis. I would say that is one of the main reasons why it
would actually be difficult for us to work alongside them. There can be
dialogue but not cooperation.

Few, however, were willing to be as direct as Caroline Armstrong at Grey's
Hospital, whose faith and scientific training led her to view traditional healing as
an obscurantist burden on those to whom she ministered.

I think the African people have got a long tradition of being aware of the
spiritual realm, much more than we in the West have allowed ourselves, so
there's a lot of mystical and occult stuff that goes on. One of their fundamental beliefs is the whole thing of the ancestor and placating the ancestor. All misfortunes are due to that. It's something which I believe is a
bondage. Some of those people who call themselves Christians are Christians, but they haven't relinquished, they haven't released themselves
from the bondage of what they must do, the sacrifices they must make for
their ancestors.

Just beneath the surface, there were concerns that since traditional healers
couldn't really cure their patients, the charges they made for their services bordered
on quackery and the fraudulent exploitation of the desperation of the sick. Sister
Margaret Shangase vividly recounted one such case in Pietermaritzburg.

He had these sores from head to toe, and one day he met a traditional
healer who told him that he could cure AIDS. Then this man came to
me and said, "Sister, the traditional healer is asking me to go and stay for
three months with him. He says he's definitely going to heal me of this
virus." I said to him, "All right."

Before he went to this man, he had lost a lot of weight. He was thin and
had sores all over his body. When he came back, he was so excited.
There was nothing, no sores, nothing, and he had gained a lot of weight.
And when he came in, he just hugged me and said, "I've been cured of
AIDS." I said, "Is that so?" He said, "Yes. This man is just waiting for his

money now." I said to him, "I'm happy with you, but let us go and test
your blood again." I took his blood, it was tested, and when the result came
back, the viral load was times two before he left. I took the first result, and
I showed him the second result, and he wept and wept.

In an account that had all of the features of a morality tale, Shangase then told of
how the disillusioned man turned from the false hopes of the traditional healer and
embraced Western medicine. He offered his services to her when she sought to
educate others who might be lured into spending what little they had for treatments that did not work: "When you go and talk to the young people in schools or
in the community, may I join you? I want to tell them that the virus is here to stay,
and it exists, and nobody can cure it."

Sacerdotal Medicine

Traditional healers had no monopoly on spirituality. In a striking way, many
doctors and nurses brought their Christian faith to their work with patients, at
times as a consolation to those for whom medicine could offer so little but also
for deeper religious reasons. Working in the Christian environment of McCord
Hospital, Henry Sunpath saw evangelization as central to his clinical efforts.

> I have a philosophy of life and a mindset that whenever I find a patient who
> is in bad physical health and in danger of losing his life, or one who is
> terminally ill, I take the opportunity to present the gospel of salvation
> through faith in the Lord Jesus Christ to them. It's been my practice
> from the first time I started as a doctor. I do it on a day-to-day basis
> with patients and a bit more zealously in people I know are terminally ill.
> Over the years, I have seen many people, even on their deathbeds, actu-
> ally have so much hope after putting faith in the Lord Jesus Christ, and
> that has encouraged me. It is part of my practice as a Christian and as a
> doctor to do that all the time.

But convictions like those of Sunpath could be found among caregivers in public
hospitals that were formally secular. At the Church of Scotland Hospital, a mission
hospital until 1975, François Eksteen saw in his pediatric work a duty to heal in
God's name. Deeply religious, he spoke about how he cautiously approached
spiritual matters with his patients.

> In most of my patients, I don't directly refer to Christian faith. One must be
> careful; one doesn't try to hammer the patient with theological doctrine.
> But you want to find out whether the patient does have peace with God if
> you see the patient is actually in the process of dying.

Eksteen remembered a young child, abandoned in the hospital by his family, whose life, he felt, had been touched by his decision to bring him closer to God.

I remember this child. He was very depressed. He almost never smiled, even after he had become stronger as a result of food and treatment. Eventually, he was taken by a foster mother, but his disease progressed. I remember it was about two years after we first saw him, he came in a very emaciated condition. I personally thought that this child was at the end, that this was terminal. One day, I decided I would like to take the child to our pastor, who was a Zulu man and let me pray with the boy.

With medical treatment, the child began to improve physically. As remarkable for Eksteen was the emotional transformation he witnessed.

The child started improving after about four or five weeks. He started smiling a bit. I remember the last time I saw him was about eight months ago, and by that time he was six years old, and he still had fairly good body weight. But at that time, he started to develop serious rashes. I said to him, he must trust the Lord Jesus Christ. And he must pray to him. I could see that he would do that.

Prayer could also serve to deepen a commitment to very sick patients. Sister Lulu Mtwisha, a retired nurse who had worked at Groote Schuur Hospital, spoke of a young terminal patient for whom a religious intervention was critical.

He had a few months to live. I said, "Do you want me to pray for you?" And he said, "OK, yes. I wouldn't mind." I just prayed with my heart and God understands. I felt so connected to this young man, and ultimately, I ended up adopting him. He called me Momma.

For Hannah Mothshedisi Sebitloane at King Edward VIII Hospital, it was not her inability to save the life of a dying woman that represented her failure, but rather the missed opportunity to bring her to God.

From a Christian point of view, I felt like I had failed. I felt I knew where she was going. Her life was very limited. We didn't have much that we could do for her. And I thought, from a spiritual point of view, I could have led her to the Lord and helped her to come to terms with her condition.

Even among the religious, few became as deeply involved in offering spiritual intervention as David Spencer, an infectious disease specialist who had studied at the Cleveland Clinic in the United States, who prayed with his patients, spoke in tongues, and, following the scriptural stories, washed his patients' feet.

One of my patients, a young man and university lecturer, was a hemophiliac who had HIV and died in about '98. He was admitted to the
Johannesburg Hospital a couple of years before he died. At the time, he had
a persistently high fever; the likely diagnosis was *Mycobacterium avium
intracellulare* [MAI]. Despite appropriate medication, his fever just sat up
at 40°. He was very sick. After I had completed ward rounds, I felt a
strong urge inside of me to pray with him. I went back to his bed and asked
him if I could pray with him. I recall thinking to myself that if the MAI
drugs weren't going to work, there was nothing else that we would be able
to do for him. It was in the early afternoon. Praying in front of my colleagues was for me something of a hurdle psychologically. I went back and
I said to this boy, "Can I pray with you?" And he said, "Yes." I prayed
with him. And his fever came down kind of miraculously, and he got
better.

Maybe two years later, he was dying of liver failure from his hepatitis
C virus infection. By that time, he had married. They had no kids because he was a hemophiliac and he had AIDS. And there was so much anger
and a lot of questions. "Why did I have to have hemophilia? Why did
I have to get HIV from a blood transfusion I was given? I've lived a clean
life." His wife was a bit older than he and wanted to have kids.

About two weeks before he died, he was admitted with fever, and I and
two friends went, and his wife was with him in the ward. My friends, who
I had asked to come and pray, suggested that we wash her feet and those
of her dying husband, as Jesus had once done in the Gospel. It had a
cathartic effect—because they hadn't been able to speak and say goodbye to
one another. It was all so easy. It kind of broke the ice, washing their
feet, the two of them in the same bed. And the tears just flowed, ours
and theirs, and they hugged one another. The whole issue of forgiveness
and anger over not being able to have children just came out into all of
us, like unplugging a dam, just poured out. It was an awesome evening.
I think we all felt as though we were standing on holy ground. That evening,
something happened, some job was done of healing that was profoundly
deep, healing in that marriage, healing in that boy. He didn't want to
die, but somehow he'd finally got to a place of saying, "It has to be, and
I just want to say goodbye to you. I love you." It was just very, very
awesome for me and my two friends. We were there on holy territory.

I would love to see that happening throughout this country, throughout
this nation. That out of the tragedy of the epidemic a healing comes that
is deep, tender, and enduring.

The religious faith of the devout Christian doctors served both the patients
and themselves. Compared to eternity, life was short, whatever the cause of death.
Such faith allowed Helga Holst, the medical superintendent of McCord Hospital,

among others, to maintain, in the midst of an epidemic for which treatment was limited, a perspective that forestalled depression and despair.

> As long as you are able to help a person to either accept their illness or get through its difficult aspects, you'll make a difference in that person's life. But there is a bit more to this than that. Each one of us is going to die at some point, the people with AIDS earlier than they would ordinarily. My belief system is that the life that we have on earth is limited, but it's not the end, that the end is much bigger. Eternity lies ahead of each one of us, and whether we have a couple more years here on earth or not ultimately isn't what the issue is. The issue is, where are you going to spend eternity? And if we, through the care that we give to people, can offer the hope of life in eternity, that is a worthy success and a victory.

Death's Toll

The centrality of religious convictions was all the more important because, as the AIDS epidemic began to take hold in the mid- to late 1990s, death became far more common. At Grey's Hospital, Caroline Armstrong had established close relationships with many of her patients. She noted how death had begun to define her work and recalled an experience that showed her what she might do for those whose lives were near the end.

> There are so many people who are dying. One patient, who presented in 1998 with cryptococcal meningitis, lived for many years. She was so compliant. She went on and off fluconazole. When the hospital was out of stock, she'd be off; when it was in stock, she'd be on. But she managed to pull through. I had a close relationship with her; she became a real friend. She came all the way up from Durban every month to pick up her treatment, and she was doing well. And then, at the end of 2003, she started to lose weight, and she started to become a bit deaf. She was in her right mind, but everything was just failing. She was in a wheelchair. And we used to just talk about it. I said, "How do you feel about this? How do you feel about all this fighting and your dying?" She had two children, and she said, "Well, you know, my mother's there, and she's still quite young. She's going to look after the children." We would just talk: "Do you have faith? What do you believe happens after you die? Are you frightened of that?" We'd talk about it, because it was obvious that she was going to die.

But such consolation was not always available. Laura Campbell, who had done a special diploma in palliative medicine, wept as she told of an experience that seemed to epitomize what doing AIDS work had become for her.

> We are on the wards every day. It was last week that we saw this man with
> Kaposi's sarcoma all over his legs. We tried to get him a bed at our hos-
> pice and put him on some morphine. Two days later, I go back and ask,
> "Did he get a bed at hospice?" "No, he's passed away." Every single time
> you go back to visit people, they have passed away. What's the use?

Ramesh Laloo Bhoola, after almost 30 years in private practice, also found it difficult not to sense failure in his work with AIDS patients.

> It's more difficult to get through the trauma of treating these patients and
> not winning all the time. We had control. You treated a patient with
> tuberculosis knowing he was going to get better nine times out of ten. Now
> you treat cryptococcal meningitis. You've done everything you can for
> one week; he still dies. I just ask[ed] my partner, "What else could I do?"
> He said, "Well, you've done everything you can."

His sense of powerlessness was echoed by a recent graduate from medical school
doing his mandatory community service at rural Emmaus Hospital. For him,
the repetitive experience of dealing with death had already begun to wear him
down, affecting his interest in work and medicine. "You don't want to go to work
every day because you know that someone's going to die. You become depressed,
and it's a struggle."

Even those whose experience and orientation to medicine had, they thought,
prepared them for death, found the endless succession of patients dying of AIDS
difficult to endure. Years earlier, in 1995, when Bernhard Gaede trained at McCord
Hospital, he learned how precious it could be to speak with dying patients and their
families. Of caring for a woman who had died of renal disease after he had brought
both her and her extended family to a sense of acceptance, he said, "It was really
very wonderful." Now, AIDS brought him back to his encounters as a medical
student with continuous, impersonal death in Soweto's Baragwanath Hospital.

> What I find quite difficult is that so much of death is anonymous, that
> people come in, they are moribund and die the next day. Families bring
> people in; they have got severe oral thrush and are emaciated. They have got
> severe diarrhea and three or four days later they die. It's a flood where
> it's difficult to engage with it. It blunts us to treating people very carefully.

Like Gaede, Paul Nijs too believed that the enemy was less death than the way
modern medicine managed the dying. He recalled that, at 26, with advanced
training in tropical medicine, he had his first experience with work in North Africa.

> Before I left for Algeria, I had concluded that I'm not there to prolong
> someone's life or to keep somebody here until I don't know when; that is

not really how I see health care. Health care to me is really trying to
help people and to improve their quality of life, not trying to keep them
away from death.

Working in the AIDS clinic at Edendale Hospital, he had to confront his own
deeply held beliefs. When patients died so routinely, he questioned his work as a
doctor.

I go through highs and lows. There are periods when you accept what
is happening, and then you really feel OK. You think, "Yes, I'm doing
something valuable." But there are periods when I really think that I must
get out of this now, because it damages me.

The most searing memories were of the pediatric wards that had been so
transformed by AIDS. From that experience, some drew lessons about how best to
meet the needs of dying children. To Neil McKerrow in Pietermaritzburg, the need
to comfort the suffering and dying children on his ward made it clear that there
was no alternative but to accept the inevitability of death and to do so in a way that
eased their pain.

It's walking into a ward and having 12 children in a row all emaciated or
with severe respiratory disease. But it's not going to kill them immediately.
They are going to lie there day in, day out, without significant improve-
ment. It becomes important for the younger staff to begin looking at how
we allow those children to die with dignity.
    The starting point for me is to recognize that death doesn't mean we
have failed. We have two purposes. The first is to delay the presentation
of AIDS. So we have to promote well-being and ensure that the children
have a longer healthy life. When they develop AIDS, we've got to shift
the emphasis to looking at comfort. When the children become chronically
ill, we have got to look at our role. Are we prolonging death, or are we
promoting comfort? When we start looking at dying with a bit of dignity,
the first step is to change our goals. It mustn't be to keep this child alive
at all costs, because the cost is often at the expense of the child. We are
prolonging suffering; we are prolonging the mourning process of the
parents.

Paul Roux, whose pioneering work at Groote Schuur Hospital made clear how
much could be done for very sick children with AIDS, also underscored how loving
care allowed him to let go at the end.

The worst week that I can remember, we had five children dying in the
ward. That was one every working day. It was just not that kind of ward at

all until the late 1990s. We never had death, or maybe one death every six months, from completely expected causes. Now, we were having two or three deaths a week. But it was something that we could all deal with, because we were responding to the loss of children that we had come to love in exactly the same way that we would have mourned a friend or a family member we had come to love. It was part of the mourning process that we all go through in a way to get over those losses. This is so different from the situation that happens in other hospitals within our pediatric health care service, where they don't have continuity of care. They don't get the opportunity to look after children—every child who dies there is a stranger.

Not all pediatricians could attain the relative equanimity described by Roux and McKerrow. Ashraf Coovadia, a 37-year-old pediatrician at Coronation Hospital in Johannesburg, spoke in 2003 of the desolation of mothers whose children had just died and of his own sense of loss in finding words that might offer some consolation to them. He recalled one infant sent to his hospital.

She had diarrhea and her hemoglobin was down, her white cell count was down, all the cell lines were down. When we received her, she looked very emaciated, very tiny for her age of 15 months. She came with the mother.

Over the next few days, she needed oxygen. She had severe pneumonia already and signs of AIDS dementia. It was quite obvious to us that she was in a very advanced stage of the disease. We made it clear to the mother that her prognosis wasn't very good. Over the next few days, she was actually getting worse and worse. Our policy is always to allow the parents time to be prepared for the inevitable. So we would talk to the mother and tell her that things are not going well, and the child isn't doing too well.

She put on a brave face and said, "I understand, doctor." Came the weekend, I was on call. The child was so looking like it was very near the end. We spoke to the mother again. She broke down. Our wards, unfortunately, aren't cubicalized. The mother had no privacy. Everyone around could see the kind of suffering that she was going through, with what the baby's going through. She just completely broke down and started crying. We took her to an outside room and we spoke to her. I think there are no words that you could use to console her. The child died. The father came. It's a very difficult moment for us. It's difficult.

I don't think medical school has prepared us for dealing with death. Till today, medical students aren't prepared. With children, it's even worse, because it's not meant to be that children die before their parents. There are no words that can tell the parents how I feel and console them. As a profession, doctors don't know ourselves where to turn for help. We really don't.

Even as they worked to relieve the suffering of individual children, to ease their inevitable deaths, and to comfort bereaved parents, doctors had to cope with their own growing sorrow. While some could preserve a professional and protective distance, others were deeply shaken, experiencing despair, a sense of outrage, and then an emotional blunting that revealed their own exhaustion. At King Edward VIII, Kogie Naidoo came early to AIDS in children and watched with a growing sense of dismay and alarm as the fatalities mounted.

The pediatric wards were full. The intensive care units [ICUs] were full, and the outpatients were full. You were seeing the same kids over and over again with recurrent otitis media, reactivation TB, chronic diarrhea, wasting, kwashiorkor, marasmus, all HIV positive. There is so much suffering, and you wonder, what will we have 20 years from now? Who is going to drive the economy?

You get called at midnight. The nurse will call you to say the baby is gasping, please come. You go there, and you see a nine-month-old, and you wonder, should I resuscitate? Should I give him adrenaline? What can I do? You don't really want to continue the suffering but, on the other hand, there is a mother who still wants to hold her baby for one more day.

You can see a holocaust; you can see babies dying. You wonder whether you can do something to limit this. And surely, there has to be an answer. You read in the scientific journals that great strides have been done to reduce mother-to-child transmission of HIV. You wonder, why don't these clinical trials come to South Africa? Why can't we just widen the access, so we can limit the disease that we see among the children? It is just too much. After a while, you become emotionally blunted.

I could deal with it. I had so much energy. I felt that I could make a difference, and on a day-to-day basis my task was to make somebody smile. I had boundless energy. In fact, my colleagues used to label me as being "hyperthyroid," because they used to wonder why I could never tire. But all that changed. You become weighed down and emotionally blunted. I recognized it when I had my own children, and I could not connect with them. I had to seek help, because I knew that there was something deeply wrong with me. I couldn't talk to the mothers. I could not tell them, "Your baby is not going to live the week, the diarrhea is too severe. We can't help; the pneumonia is not responding to the antibiotics." I couldn't live with myself.

In Johannesburg, Dalu Ndiweni was struck by how many did not understand how profound an effect the care of dying children had on doctors.

Many doctors say, "I can't continue like that. I can't see babies dying."
Stunningly enough, that's why maybe some doctors are afraid of children.
People think that doctors get used to people dying. Amazing. You wax
and wane. Sometimes you feel much more vulnerable than other times. It
leaves you exhausted.

The experience of caregivers like Naidoo compelled those who worked with
children to consider how close they could permit themselves to get to those whose
prospects were so dismal. Clarence Mini, committed to AIDS care since his return
from exile in 1990, recalled a clinical encounter where his efforts to remain professionally detached had failed.

One granny came to me with her four-year-old granddaughter. She had
chronic otitis media and the ears are oozing pus and the eyes are looking
strange, according to the granny. She said, "You know, doctor, I go to
the clinic, they give me the eye drops and something for the ears, but what
I can't take is that in the middle of the night, this baby stands up on the
bed and she screams. She has got pain all over her body, she gets fever, the
temperature goes literally through the roof, she burns with this temperature." And she said, what really touched me, "When God took away my
daughter, I said to him, please Lord, let me keep this grandchild, and
this grandchild is my consolation. I see her mother in her. And now God
does this to me, letting this child go through this suffering. What am
I supposed to do?" As a doctor, you do your best to detach yourself from
this suffering to be able to work and help others, and you've got to be
strong. You don't want to give in.

In this case, he was overwhelmed by the grandmother's anguish. Years later, he still
had trouble speaking of the event without weeping because it still evoked in him
such profound sadness.

Those who worked with adults also found it necessary to establish a professional distance that was protective but which did not compromise their abilities to
meet their patients' needs. Knowing that he could pull back or flee when the price
he had to pay became more than he could bear allowed Bongani Thembela, a
veteran of public hospitals and private practice, to remain open to the suffering
that greater intimacy entailed.

I tend to interact with my patients. I think I have a good habit, which I also
tell students is a bad habit, that sometimes I get too much involved with
my patients. Generally speaking—I'm a Zulu myself—Zulu men tend not
to want to show their emotions in public. I think I'm one of those that
you call a "sissy." I can remember many times sitting at the AIDS clinic at
Edendale with a patient, and the two of us are crying. Maybe I start crying

first, maybe they start crying first for various reasons, some at the time their
disease is diagnosed, some of them when they see that things are not
looking up.

If I have patients whom I'm going to be seeing over a long period of
time, I tend to want to know where they stay, who the parents are, etc.
I get involved in that sort of thing over and above the medical things.
I think that's the key. But I also have an escape valve where I know that
tomorrow, if I decide this is enough for me, I'll open a private practice.
It helps me to know that I can walk away from this any time without ma-
jor disruptions in my personal life. But I cannot say the same for everyone.
I know it's hard on them.

Others found alternative ways to preserve emotional distance, both to protect
themselves and because they believed it was essential to do so to enhance their
capacity to work effectively. "For you to continue, somehow you need to take it out
of your mind as fast as possible, because someone else in the same family needs
you," said Musa Gumede at his private office in Durban. Gumede, who had been
born in a Black township on the outskirts of that city in 1968, spoke of his anger.
"You're sad, but soon you need to take it out of your head. Otherwise, it will engulf
you and consume you."

The structure of the health care system, its burdens and demands, as well as the
way physicians chose to pursue their professional work within such constraints,
made it possible for some to work with dying patients without being emotionally
worn down. Both a clinician and an administrator in Pietermaritzburg, James
Muller defined his role in a way that shielded him from the emotional toll he might
otherwise have experienced.

I found that I had a lot more difficulty dealing with death and issues
relating to death when I was working in Canada, because you were much
more directly involved with the patient and the family. You had to try to
confront it yourself. You had to try to help them to confront it. Here,
you do not do that as a physician. It tends not to be part of your job,
particularly at a place like Edendale. You administer the treatment. You do
your best that you can for the patient. Then, if the patient dies, you move
on to the next case. You tend not to be directly involved in trying to
help the family to come to terms with it and to develop some kind of an
understanding of why it should have happened to their relatives. One of the
things I always found very difficult, and I still do, is confronting and
interacting with people when I know that they are dying and they know
they are dying. I've never really come to grips with that.

Among the strategies available to doctors as they struggled with the emotional
impact of clinical work was to devote themselves to research. Such efforts at once

represented an effort to expand the range of clinical possibilities and also reduced the intensity of direct patient exposure. Anisa Mosam, who, as a dermatologist, never expected to see many of her patients die, felt she had no alternative but to engage in clinical studies if she were to continue her AIDS work.

> Kaposi's sarcoma is one of the most devastating conditions you have seen here with HIV. I have seen young patients coming in with these huge legs or with lesions on their faces. It's absolutely disfiguring. They can't swallow. They can't see. They can't walk. They are bedridden. I got tired of saying to patients, "We can't do anything for you. This is what it is. This is what you have. You have probably got six months to live." So I felt, if I don't do something, I am really just not going to survive in this set-up. I am going to leave here, or I am just going to end up feeling like I am not really doing much.

At Baragwanath, Glenda Gray, whose work on preventing mother-to-child transmission of HIV would give her the opportunity to act both as a scientist and as a politically engaged physician to save newborns from HIV infection, spoke of how she had been transformed by seeing so many sick children.

> It was very hard. These children, earlier on, I knew personally and individually. And I just saw the distress in those women and how hard they tried not for this to happen. In the beginning, you are outraged that children are dying from this disease. You get to a stage where you go into overload. You block it out. You are seeing so many deaths, this is just normal. You forget that children live and get over illnesses, and accept that kids just die with this disease. And that is what's horrible, because you've become desensitized.

While her capacity for outrage drew her to research—she had gone to New York to study epidemiology—her research in turn protected her from the emotional blunting that she saw in others and that was beginning to affect her as well: "Maybe it was easier because we had pulled out of service and become researchers. There was a time when I was a treater and a researcher, and then I got enough funding to become just a researcher."

Others faced the bleak picture by fashioning new clinical programs that could affect the lives of their very sick patients. If they could not prevent the inevitability of death, they could at least regain a modicum of professional resilience. Tony Moll did just that at the Church of Scotland Hospital.

> Deaths of the young were becoming a common thing. I could see that this can potentially demoralize staff. It can create a sense of helplessness in the hospital. Very early on, we tackled this head on by saying that we, as

doctors, are going to set an example, that whatever condition the patient comes in with, we are going to go all out and help, admit, and treat with whatever we can. What we can do is give social support, give encouragement. And that has kept us going.

But despite his fortitude and an almost relentless optimism, his spirit would at times fail him. Then, he would turn to his wife and his faith.

I have many times gone home and said, "I can't handle this any more. I would like to, but I don't have the inner strength any more. I feel that I am burning out, that the duties and the workload is just overwhelming." There were strategies that we came up with. One was to have a little prayer meeting every morning amongst ourselves as doctors. Before the prayer meeting, we would talk about our immediate burdens, pray about it together, and then go into the day's work.

For Sue Roberts, with years of nursing experience at Johannesburg's Helen Joseph Hospital, it was the knowledge that she had not only comforted patients but empowered them that made the years of dealing with dying patients more bearable.

We have had patients who, when we've first met them, hadn't come to terms with their HIV, hadn't come to terms with themselves. And they managed to disclose to their family, managed to make plans and to get themselves identity books so that they know that they can be buried. A lot of our patients have actually also become activists. To see the growth in them is extremely satisfying. Yes, they may eventually die, but they've managed to contribute in a way that they never would have contributed without the HIV, and I think that's a consolation.

But however they worked to shield themselves, however much they understood the importance of retaining the ability to meet the needs of their patients, the emotional toll exacted by the magnitude of the epidemic, the limits of clinical intervention, and the death-defining aspect of their work had a crushing impact on some doctors, even as they carried on. Recalling the late 1990s at Edendale Hospital, Neil McKerrow said of the senior physicians:

I don't know whether it was the disintegration of the hospital that had once been so good, or working in that environment filled with so many constraints, or if it was the nature of the clinical work, but depression amongst the senior staff was a major problem.

Bernhard Gaede, whose work at rural Emmaus Hospital was especially difficult because of chronic staff shortages, gave voice to the frustration and despair he felt when his emotional reserves had been all but exhausted.

I can feel when I'm getting closer to burn[ing] out, when that blunting just
becomes worse and worse and worse. You don't want to engage with it,
because engaging with it makes you tired, makes you exhausted. You've
just heard it so many times, and it's not interesting any more. You don't
want to know about another person's pain any more. I can't remember the
patient's name; I can't remember where they come from. Often, two
o'clock in the morning, when you are tired, they would come. This person has been like this for how long, and now you come at two in the morning? I mean, why are you wasting my time? It becomes very difficult then
to start to say, "So what does it feel like?" Actually, I don't care. I don't
give a fuck. I don't want to engage with it.

And, however hard doctors worked, it was nurses who bore the brunt of the
added burden. The apparent futility of care and the fact that they were increasingly
required to clean patients who could not control their bowels made many re-
sentful. Sue Roberts explained the discontent. "They are now dealing with patients
that are sick, and they really can't make a difference. Why should they be there?"
Laura Campbell had witnessed the kind of outburst such resentment could pro-
voke.

The nurse in charge said that you have to get these patients out. She said,
"We can't nurse them; we are not nurses any more. We are just cleaning up
diarrhea and feeding people." So I think that they're getting frustrated,
because they are not able to nurse any more.

Glenda Gray noted how the anger of nurses played out at Baragwanath
Hospital. Some, she observed, "have just given up; like a lot of civil servants, they
have given up." Among the most empathetic, rage served to fuel a process of
politicization. They would eventually join community activists and doctors in the
emergent movement demanding better conditions for themselves and their patients, as well as access to antiretroviral therapies. Most lived with their anger.

They are angry because of the increase of the workload, which is not getting better. They are angry because they are from the same community
as the patients, and they themselves are vulnerable, as well as also probably
having to deal with HIV within themselves and their families. And they
have no support.

4

Limited Access

As the number of critically ill AIDS patients seeking hospital care mounted, the capacity of already strained institutions to respond eroded. Describing Baragwanath Hospital, Haroon Saloojee, who over time had shifted his focus from neonatal care to broad concerns about health policy, observed, "The situation has changed, mainly related to HIV. There is this enormous stress on beds. The only way you respond to that is turn people away. So you only admit the very sick."

But although necessary, turning people away was not so easy. Triage inevitably posed moral quandaries. In Johannesburg, Pinky Ngcakani, who by 2004 had left work in a public hospital out of sheer frustration, described the dilemmas she had previously faced in deciding whom to admit when her hospital was already full.

> So it was looking at the patients and then deciding who is sicker than
> the other; who can I admit and who can I not? And you knew that the
> ones that would not be admitted were going to be back a day or two later,
> because they should have been admitted, but I didn't have the space avail-
> able. And how can you say, Really this one has chronic diarrhea and is
> dehydrated, and I cannot admit her; that one has meningitis, and he
> needs more help. So they stayed in casualty overnight, or over two
> days, whilst waiting for an available bed.

Overcrowded tertiary care institutions, whose outpatient clinics and wards were filled to capacity, sought to shift their patients to other health care settings. Bureaucratic rigidities served to hold demand at bay. Themba Mabaso, a private practitioner in Durban, sardonically recounted the treatment to which he and a patient had been subjected.

> I had a terrible situation where I sent a patient to King Edward VIII
> with a specimen bottle. He phoned to say that he had been sent away
> and told to go to another hospital. I told him to wait for me there, where

I explained to the nurse who was doing the sorting that in Mahatma
Gandhi Hospital, there is no urologist, and this particular problem needs
a urologist. The nurse refused. She showed me a chart which showed
that if you live in this area, you go to that hospital. She said, "Now
you've driven here, you can drive him to Mahatma Gandhi. Ask the doctor
there to write a letter and bring him back. Then, I'll take him."

Describing the plight of those who needed inpatient care, Mabaso was even
more bitter.

There is no place for people who are dying of HIV in hospitals. If
we send them to King Edward VIII in respiratory distress, they are going
to die on the bench waiting to see a doctor. If they do get admitted for
cryptococcal meningitis, they may be shunted to an inferior hospital
after 72 hours. You don't even have clinics in those hospitals. It's just
the ward where some of the most incompetent nurses or people who
are tired of working go and spend their last days of work. You send
someone there, and they are going to die there, or they may send
them home to die.

Some hospitals were compelled to adopt measures that represented a throw-
back to what had, at times, been necessary in Black hospitals during the apartheid
era. At the Church of Scotland Hospital, with 350 official beds, Tony Moll told of
his strategy to make room in his already filled medical wards and the institutional
resistance his efforts provoked.

We began using what we call "floor beds," which are blankets rolled
out under the bed of another patient or between two beds. The patients
were quite happy to accept this. What happened then was the management of the district came back to us, and said, "We see that you've got
more than 100 percent occupancy of your beds. How does this work? We
can't have more than one person in a bed." We said that we were using
floor beds. They said, "Well, the computer cannot accept this. There is
no block to fill in the statistic for floor beds." So they actually prohibited us
from making such accommodations. If we are on duty 9, 10, 11 o'clock
at night, and a patient comes in and the ward is full, we have to admit that patient, put up a drip and initiate antibiotics. And what we
have had to do now is to put the patient on a trolley and let them
wait outside in a passage until a bed becomes available. And this is an
every night's story.

Despite the existence of triage mechanisms that sought to limit admissions
of those who were too sick to benefit from care, and despite the reliance on

bureaucratic roadblocks to restrict the number of AIDS patients that could be admitted, those with HIV-related conditions began to displace other sick patients. "The Impact of HIV/AIDS on the Health Sector," a report prepared for the national Department of Health in 2003, noted that as the epidemic increased, those with HIV had begun to "crowd out" others deemed to be less needy.[1] Commenting on this phenomenon at his own hospital, Tony Moll said:

> Terminally ill AIDS patients can be so sick with fulminating PCP or cryptococcal meningitis, or have a very bad infected wound, that we try to give them priority over a diabetic or hypertensive that might not be so sick. They are ambulatory people and can be treated at home.

Home-Based Care

With hospitals filled beyond capacity and patients desperate for medical services, a few doctors and nurses developed innovative approaches to treatment. These services were often organized without financial or political support from the provincial Departments of Health, and used whatever resources could be garnered. In Tugela Ferry, for example, Tony Moll and his staff sought to extend their strained resources by introducing home-based care.

> I can remember in 1997, we would be admitting a few AIDS patients every day. At the same time, we were looking at the provincial Department of Health, waiting for a plan of action for managing this epidemic. But very soon we realized that there was no such thing. At that time, there was this poisonous attitude amongst doctors and nurses, who would say to the patient, "I am sorry; we see that you have AIDS. There is nothing more that we can do for you. Let me give you some tablets to take home, and when you have a problem, come back again." And we realized, as doctors, surely there is something that we can do, surely there is some structure of support that we can offer these patients. It was in that environment that we came across the concept of home-based care, because we could see that our resources within the hospital were completely limited.

In Durban, Moll found a training program "where semiliterate people were being taught to care for dying patients in their own homes." Inspired by what he had seen, he sought out volunteers in his own community.

> In the beginning, we went to churches, we went to shops, we went to school principals, we went to key community figures, *ndunas*, or chiefs of the area. We actually knocked on doors, went into huts, sat alongside women

or men in the community, and said, "This is what we are looking for; are you willing to volunteer?" The response was overwhelming, because here was something that we were offering to a community that had already experienced the hopelessness of HIV/AIDS. So our problem wasn't recruiting, but selecting from people who were willing to come forward.

But if he uncovered a wellspring of good will in his community, he also encountered resistance, not only from his own nurses, but from representatives of the local health bureaucracy as well.

There was a nurse who had the job of what they called TB coordinator, and this nurse reported back to TB coordinators of the whole district together, and I went along to some of their meetings. We announced that we were starting a home-based care program, and everybody said no, this is not official government policy; there are no written documents concerning who must do it, job descriptions, or anything like that. We can't get involved. They weren't interested.

Despite such resistance, Moll pressed ahead. The program, which began in December 1997, captured the energy and imagination of the Tugela Ferry community, which made it its own. At the outset there were 20 volunteers,

semiliterate people living in our community. Some of them are housewives and some of them are people who own small businesses or are selling vegetables as vendors. Basically, we were looking for respected, credible, trusted people in the community that could join us.

By 2004, the Tugela Ferry program involved more than 200 care providers "who are like partners in a community. It's like having an extended ward out of the hospital. Our home-based carers act as nurses." The volunteers visited patients once or twice a week. If it seemed that a social worker was necessary, that could be arranged. If the patient needed a hospital readmission, the volunteer would take the required first steps. "This became a kind of safety net, becoming a huge important resource out there." Most impressive to Moll himself was that

the program is running by itself, and it's unbelievable. What is actually happening is that the home-based carers are selecting and recruiting their own volunteers in the community and helpers to come along. They have on their own been mentoring other community members in what to do and how to do it in such a way now that our training program is self-perpetuated.

At Mosvold, an isolated hospital near the Mozambique border, Ann Barnard, who, since the age of 12, had wanted to work in Africa "to work in a developing world situation," initiated a home care program involving a small, committed group of 12 workers, who were able to penetrate remote areas whose populations lacked health services and to provide families with medicines, education, and social support.

> Just visiting and showing that they care seems to make a huge differ-
> ence. We have seen people who have really lost hope and taken to their
> beds. And when the home-based care team gets involved, patients of-
> ten walk within a couple of weeks.
> They are really there to try and support the families. They teach
> the families how to care for the patients, how to turn them and do bed
> baths, how to apply dressings and control their pain and diarrhea. The
> nurse is able to get drugs out to patients, just basics like fluconazole
> and Bactrim, and more complex drugs like morphine for the terminally
> ill ones. There were whole loads of people in the community who just
> weren't getting any sort of health care service; they just couldn't access it.

With support from the Elton John Foundation, Barnard was able to pay those who provided home-based care. In fact, she believed it was wrong to depend on volunteers for such work. "I didn't feel that it's fair to expect people to do such a job as volunteers. There is such huge poverty in the area; we can't ask people to volunteer. It wasn't very much; we were only giving 800 rand a month."

Rationing Care in the Public Sector: Resource Limitations or Discrimination?

However much home-based care helped to limit the burden on hospitals and clinics in the public sector, clinicians recognized that they would have to continue to care for people in an environment of chronic resource deprivation. Material limits virtually defined medical practice and helped to set the rules for care. The acceptance of privation and of the need to maximize available resources was an integral part of the professional culture, even before AIDS began to exacerbate the situation. Reflecting both resignation and a pragmatic determination in the face of scarcity, the medical manager of Emmaus Hospital, Bernhard Gaede, observed, "I have always worked in a framework where I assume that there aren't enough resources. For me, it has always been, OK, how can we find a solution, rather than becoming indignant."

Given the scarcity that defined their world, even those deeply committed to the care of their patients could embrace the rationing of services as a moral imperative.

For Haroon Saloojee—who would become an expert witness for the plaintiffs in a successful suit forcing the government of President Thabo Mbeki to provide antiretrovirals to pregnant women—deciding who would have access to limited resources was both necessary and routine.

> I believe that my role as a citizen of the community is to ensure the
> best utilization of resources. So it may not make sense to continue offering
> a baby care for five days instead of two days. Maybe the baby might
> have shown improvement after three or five days, but I'd rather have
> those three days for another baby who has a better chance. I was never
> uncomfortable with this, because we were often turning away babies, good,
> strong, big babies who only needed one day of the intensive care unit,
> simply because we didn't have the beds. Occasionally, those babies died
> in our wards. That kind of balancing act, I got into that role fairly
> comfortably. I hope I got the balance right; one never knows. We tried
> to make it as systematic and objective as possible.

Saloojee spoke frankly of his conversations with parents at Baragwanath Hospital concerning the resources that could be dedicated to their children and of their acquiescence to his judgments. "There was an issue of premature and low-birthweight babies," he remembered. "I was dealing with this on a daily basis. I was very straightforward with parents." He explained that if the baby made no progress, he had no alternative but to end care. There was no need to confront parents with a series of medical options. "It was a matter of fact. We are doing this. I think most parents will accept that," he said, "because in the kind of environment we worked in, the doctor was God."

This, then, was the context within which the limits imposed on care for AIDS patients occurred. At a time when the understanding of the prognosis of children with AIDS was still evolving, when the available evidence was sparse, hospitals began to lay down restrictions. Saloojee explained how the need to limit care generated action rules and remarkably little dispute.

> There wasn't a lot of debate on this issue, because people really didn't know
> how to deal with this. We had no precedent. We had a few cases of se-
> vere cancer but never on this scale. Nobody knew whether you should treat
> AIDS-related disorders twice, thrice, four times, where you draw the line.
> It was clearly perplexing to all of us not to know what we were doing.
> Where you draw the line wasn't a discussion going on in developed
> countries. So, when solutions were offered, for example, by our inten-
> sive care units, they said that the prognosis of kids admitted to the ICU was
> very poor and that 90-plus percent died. We accepted that information
> very quickly, along with the argument that kids with HIV should not
> get ICU care. There wasn't intense arguments and fights. It was, OK,

so that's the prognosis, all right, fine. Anecdote and experiential evidence quickly became translated into informal policy at the hospital level.

In 2003, Gary Maartens, 47 years old and long dedicated to providing treatment to those with HIV, expressed his support for rule-bound rationing. He defended the explicit decision of the Groote Schuur Hospital to bar AIDS patients from its ICU.

> Our intensive care unit has now made an explicit policy that they
> will not admit HIV positive people with *Pneumocystis* pneumonia
> into the ICU. I think that's not unreasonable, given that they have very
> limited facilities. The ICU doctors had looked at the mortality rates
> of the other diseases they admit to ICU; they are around 20 percent.
> They'd looked at their own *Pneumocystis* experience, and it's around
> 60 percent. That's not a good use of resources. So they have decided to
> exclude that group of patients, and I don't have a problem with that as
> long as it's explicit. I quite like that very recent trend in rationing that
> we have now.

For Maartens, it was nevertheless important to distinguish between the imposition of such limits and discriminatory practices that were injurious and unfair to people with HIV. While he had succeeded in crafting practices for his hospital that assured them access to surgical services that might have been barred to them in other institutions, he was compelled to acknowledge that resources were not equitably applied at Groote Schuur.

> AIDS, it's not like other diseases. This hospital does cardiac, liver, renal,
> bone marrow transplants. We use almost all the drugs that you would
> in the United States to prevent rejection. We do dialysis. So, expen-
> sive therapies are available here, but not for HIV. So there's that injus-
> tice; that is very hard.

It was precisely the extent to which the careful husbanding of resources could serve as a pretext for prejudicial acts that was so disturbing. In language that recalled the experience of doctors who had treated AIDS in gay men a decade earlier, Dalu Ndiweni spoke with despair about the motives of his colleagues at Johannesburg Hospital, as they made decisions involving matters of life and death.

> There is an antibiotic or drug usage committee that sits, and you say,
> "Look, this is a child who has got AIDS, and I would like to use some of the
> antibiotics that we use for severe infections." Because you could not claim
> that next week the patient would not be back with the same infection, it
> felt like you were pouring money down the drain. Our budgets are not

limitless. So because of that, discrimination against the patient with
HIV started: you could not use this drug because you're HIV positive,
because there's no hope. But you will find no one writes in black
and white that you cannot give antibiotics.

Of those who could so swiftly deny a child access to lifesaving medications, he said,
"You are trying to make yourself God. You have decided this one is going to die."

As the number of AIDS patients multiplied and as the deepening experience of
clinicians began to permit nuanced determinations about the prospects of those
infected with HIV, even those who were, in principle, committed to rationing
became increasingly troubled. It became clear to them that decisions could be
made in utter disregard for prognosis. In 2003, Ashraf Coovadia, whose interest in
palliative care made him sensitive to the need for protocols governing decisions to
withdraw treatment, was highly critical of the implicit rules governing intensive
care in his province.

A child comes in very severely distressed; if it is HIV positive, that
child won't go to an ICU. That is a rule right across at least Gauteng
Province, and I think most provinces. That is a difficult one for us to
deal with, because we argue that HIV shouldn't be looked upon as a
uniform diagnosis, with everyone having the same degree of illness. For
those children at death's door, it's defensible for them not to end up
in the ICU unit because of the futility of the treatment. The child who
has just become infected may be very healthy. But the ICU's policies
throughout the country are to exempt them from care, just as it is a
rule that no newborn under a kilogram will get ventilated. It is an
arbitrary decision. It's an unwritten law, but it's followed by all
the hospitals.

As a mother and doctor, Kogie Naidoo felt demoralized as she confronted the
intransigence of those who managed the ICU at King Edward VIII Hospital.

You work so hard to get to a point, and then all of a sudden you are
just dropping this case because there is nothing you can do. And yet, it
may be a precious baby. It may be a child after eight years of infertility. It
may be the third child and the other two have succumbed to HIV, and
you want to keep this baby alive longer for a mother whose arms are empty.
So you feel hopeless; you feel helpless. You just basically want to tell
the parents and run away so you don't have to deal with it.

Such rationing policies were not limited to the intensive care unit. Tammy
Meyers, head of the pediatric AIDS unit at Baragwanath Hospital, reported similar
struggles to get a patient admitted to the oncology service.

I remember we had a child who came in, a 10- or 11-year-old boy who came
in with a first presentation of a tumor, and I sent him down to the oncology wards. They asked me, "Has he got HIV? We can't really do anything for him." I said, "But, he's well." We actually had a CD4 count
on him which was really good; he was really well. And they said, "He's got
HIV. We can't do anything for him. If we treat him, he's going to die
anyway." I said, "This is wrong." We had a whole panel discussion around
this patient; I brought ethicists. They brought their specialists, hematolo-
gists, oncologists who said that, according to the literature, all cases of
children with cancer and HIV have died.

Ironically, despite the dire prognosis by the oncologists, the child went into re-
mission after nothing more than radiation treatment designed to provide palli-
ation.

In time, it became increasingly clear that the solution to rationing, implicit or
explicit, had to lie in a systemic change that would, paradoxically, justify more
rather than less care. James McIntyre, who knew that children with HIV at Baragwanath Hospital were "getting less care, were being discharged earlier," would
join the ranks of activists arguing for antiretroviral treatment.

I think that rationing is the wrong decision. But I think the solution to the
problem is not going to come from individual doctors or individual
hospitals. It's going to come from a policy that provides comprehensive
AIDS care as it should be provided. Doctors don't have the resources, they
don't have the drugs.

Dalu Ndiweni, who in early 2004 had just begun to use antiretrovirals on a
very limited basis, observed that the addition of such drugs spoke directly to the
nihilism that reinforced the arguments for rationing.

Our limited experience with antiretrovirals is that the children have
actually done very well. That's why we feel emotionally charged about
not doing anything. Because if the child was on antiretrovirals, people
wouldn't be saying, "Don't use antibiotics on such patients." And even the
doubting Thomases would begin to say, "Well, maybe we should do
something."

Antiretroviral Therapy: Worlds Apart

In the mid-1990s, when the HIV epidemic began its catastrophic escalation in
South Africa but when the number of clinical cases was still relatively small, the
global picture for AIDS treatment was uniformly grim. The Concorde clinical trial

in Europe in 1993 had demonstrated that AZT, the first antiretroviral drug used in the AIDS epidemic, was relatively ineffective. Then, a common bond united the richest and poorest nations. In neither was it possible to combat the underlying cause of the cascade of diseases that afflicted people with AIDS.

Remarkable changes began in 1994, when a clinical trial in the United States involving pregnant women demonstrated that the use of AZT during the second and third trimesters, and during delivery, and then administered to the newborn during the first six months of life could radically reduce the rate of maternal-fetal HIV transmission. In 1995 there was even more striking news. The first reports appeared about a new class of drugs—the protease inhibitors—which showed dramatic therapeutic efficacy when used in combination with two other antiretroviral medications. Previously measurable HIV in the blood could be reduced to undetectable levels. Some began to speak about the possibility of eliminating HIV from infected individuals. By 1996, an air of triumphalism characterized the biennial international AIDS conference in Vancouver. In countries where these drugs were available, patients were snatched back from the edge of death. But such therapies were extraordinarily costly. And thus did a global divide begin to define the AIDS pandemic. In rich nations, AIDS was increasingly viewed as a manageable, chronic, if still ultimately fatal disease. In the world's poorest nations, where the epidemic's human toll dwarfed the burden in the industrialized world, these therapies were all but inaccessible. Reflecting on what he had seen on the children's wards of Baragwanath Hospital in the 1990s, Haroon Saloojee said:

> We went through wards each day with a sense of despair—but also a sense
> that there was work to be done. These kids needed care, and we would
> do what we could, recognizing that we had seen these kids two weeks
> ago. The cure for AIDS lay beyond us.

For Steven Miller, who had been involved in treating AIDS in gay men since the 1980s and who had begun to develop an immense AIDS practice in Johannesburg, the conference reports produced a sense of

> disbelief, largely the feeling that it's just one way that we are trying to
> pacify ourselves. I think there was great skepticism about it, being very
> cautious in interpreting extremely optimistic data. I think that what
> got it to fall into place was that the pathogenesis of HIV was becoming
> a lot clearer. For the first time, we'd got some antiviral drugs that work. I
> can't say I had this sense of jubilation. It was just that feeling of exhausted
> relief.

Dennis Sifris, like Miller a gay man who had witnessed the toll taken by AIDS on his community in Johannesburg, was less restrained. He began to prescribe the new combination therapies to his private patients "as soon as we could get supplies, probably about three months after coming back from Vancouver. It was the most wonderful feeling. Suddenly, you have this wonderful drug, the best thing on the market, the triple cocktail, the miracle."

In Pietermaritzburg, Jeanne Dixon, whose commitment to meeting the needs of people with AIDS had brought her into conflict with hospital administrators, received the news very differently than did those gay doctors in private practice. Acutely aware of the poverty of those she saw, she recalled, "At that time, I was so overcome with my patients starving that I would rather have been able to feed them. It was such a remote possibility of ever being able to offer those new drugs."

But even in the relatively privileged settings within which Miller and Sifris practiced, the cost of the new medications represented a significant hurdle. Steven Miller remembered:

In those days, the cost of drugs was about 3500 rand a month, which is probably more than most persons' total salary. So we had a subgroup of wealthy people who were staying well. And they were the haves. We still had this big stream of the have-nots.

A dramatic shift occurred in 1998, when medical aid schemes, medical insurance plans that covered many employed individuals in the private and public sectors—but only 18 percent of the South African population—began to cover antiretroviral treatment. Miller and others had pressed the insurance schemes because coverage was so critical for their patients. In so doing, they had appealed to corporate self-interest.

Health insurers were starting to see how much they were spending on unnecessary illness. People would become sick. None of us would disclose the diagnosis, because we felt that there is no point in prejudicing the patient's situation. So they had these huge bills for pneumonia or meningitis. I think they started to realize that what we were saying is true. You think you are not paying for AIDS. You are, and you're actually paying more than you should. So be sensible and just redeploy the cash in a slightly different way.

In Miller's own practice, which had 1,900 patients by 2003, a drop in drug prices over time to 700–800 rand a month permitted him to put together a clinical package, including laboratory tests and office consultations, for something approximating 12,000 rand a year. He knew that such fees placed his skills and services beyond the reach of most. Making the transition to a fee schedule that effectively barred life-saving treatment from the vast numbers of men, women, and children who needed it "hurt at first." Recalling his activities during the 1980s, when AIDS struck the gay community, he believed that the current situation justified a very different approach.

I think there was a great indulgence in luxury in those terrible days of the
1980s, because all of us who were doing this work had other sources of
income. So we could give freely and generously. It's very difficult making
the transition from that to a fee-for-service situation. But I think in
time, what one comes to realize is that you can't solve the entire problem.
And if we are making things better for 1,900 people, there is actually
nothing wrong with that, because those people wouldn't have benefited
if we weren't around. The only way you can do that and keep going
is to do it on a fee-for-service basis.

David Johnson, another gay physician in Johannesburg, came to accept the
consequences of a private practice—purchased in 1994—that barred access to those
without resources from receiving anything more than his skilled clinical management.

I've had to do a serious mental readjustment on that. I've had to say to
myself that I don't have endless money. So I can't just find it and give
it to them. I do the best with what resources they have. I give them comfort and as good health as they can enjoy, and I give them dignity. That
may not be enough, but that is adequate.

Given the logic of private practice and the cost of antiretrovirals, Dennis Sifris
felt that he had no alternative but to keep those who could not afford his services
from his office. Sometimes his efforts failed, and then he was confronted with the
need to turn them away.

In private practice, the ones who come to see me can usually afford it except
the odd ones who find their way to me. They bring their children in,
who were discharged from hospital and they can't walk from the car. They
expect me to perform a miracle. You describe the cost of drugs, and
then they say, "Oh well. I've got 4 rand"; the other one says she's got 10.
And they'll get 14 rand from auntie. It's a hard thing in private practice to
say to these people, "Look, I'm sorry, I can't help you."

David Spencer, who had treated gay men at the public Johannesburg Hospital,
sought to confront the moral quandaries of caring only for those who could afford
it. At the same time, he had to face the precarious economics of his private practice.
He chose to offer discounted services one day a week.

When I moved into private practice, I wasn't making money. I said to my
financial adviser, "I want to be able to see ordinary people, not just the
wealthy." And he said, "Why don't you have a day in the week when you
charge half price? You limit it to a half an hour to bring the person in,

sort out what the problem is as quickly as you can. Then they can have access to you." That became a community day. Most of the domestic workers see me then. My major problem there is when such a patient requires hospitalization. Private hospital costs are exorbitant, and many employers cannot afford these expenses. I will write them a letter and send them through to the government hospitals, either for them to be taken over entirely and go into their AIDS clinics or for the opportunistic disease to be managed, after which they come back to me.

Spencer acknowledged in 2004 that not many of his patients were seen under his discounted plan, "only about 20 percent." When the government began to roll out its antiretroviral treatment program at the end of 2004, he brought this effort to a close.

For each of these four doctors with very restricted private practices, AIDS underwent a fundamental transformation in their patients because of the new antiretroviral cocktails. Their own clinical experiences were also radically changed. Certainly, there would be setbacks associated with the use of these drugs, side effects that could be debilitating, that required a change in regimen, or the more dramatic reconstitution syndrome, in which patients would experience severe clinical crises just as their immune systems were beginning to rebound. But AIDS was no longer a disease that promised certain death after a course of repeated bouts with life-threatening opportunistic illnesses.

Steven Miller underscored how things had changed. "The first to go was CMV retinitis, which could render people blind. People weren't getting CD4 counts that fell to zero." Speaking in 2004, he remarked, "To some extent, medicine has become terribly boring because it's 'I'm fine, the dog is fine, the cat's fine.' " The most striking contrast between Miller's world of AIDS care and that which characterized the vast untreated epidemic in South Africa was captured in his observation, "I haven't had anyone die in the last six months."

For those who worked in less restrictive private settings, whose general practice was not so dominated by AIDS and who saw patients with much more limited resources, it became necessary to engage in often difficult discussions about what they could afford to pay for treatment. Such conversations were not new to South Africa. Nor were they restricted to situations that involved AIDS. When he was at McCord Hospital, which charged for its services, Bernhard Gaede had to face such situations repeatedly. As a consequence, he came to understand the ways in which the poverty of his patients had to shape his work as a doctor.

Initially, when I started asking patients about their resources, I didn't like it at all, because it felt like it was interfering with my clinical judgment. When I looked at that reaction, I realized that part of it was that I'm scared to engage with the poverty of people. And once I realized that, I began to search for other solutions.

The life-and-death implications of such decisions in the context of AIDS made them especially difficult. Themba Mabaso recalled the impact of his patients' inability to pay for antiretroviral medications before medical insurance provided coverage in 1998 and the consequences for those lacking coverage even after such protection became available.

> There was no way you could do anything before the medical aid schemes paid for treatment. It was impossible. Even those patients who said they could pay cash didn't understand the impact of having to pay. It was like a mortgage. It used to be about 2,000 rand a month. They never understood the impact if, in the fourth month, something happened that they couldn't afford the treatment. Obviously, if they came back later and asked me for a prescription, they'd have developed resistance to the drugs.

And for his many patients who lacked medical insurance, there was little he could do. "There's a double standard here. People who are on medical aid get the better treatment; that's just the fact of life here." The stark choices that could be presented under such circumstances were not lost on Musa Gumede, who as a young man had been involved in anti-apartheid youth activities. Not infrequently, he would see couples, both of whom were infected: "Sometimes, they come together; the husband is on medical aid and the wife is not. I've got to tell one I can't give you drugs. I can't put you on. You feel useless. It's like deciding who lives and who doesn't live within the family. It's quite tough."

For those without medical insurance, physicians were forced into the uncomfortable position of having to gauge what each patient could afford. At McCord Hospital, Jane Hampton described a torturous effort to plumb her patient's finances.

> It is very difficult. You don't want to miss someone who could afford antiretrovirals. And you do not know if there is someone who might have an uncle or if the family might be able to rustle up the money. I always say in the beginning, "It is very expensive, and most people can't afford it." That's how I start. So, at the very beginning, they don't have this hope, this total hope. There was this girl. We talked about it. She said she could not afford it, and she cried. You sit there, and you can just cry with them, because there is nothing I can really do.

She understood all too well what being able to do "nothing" meant.

> It is very hard when you know that there are people that do get good care. People who can afford antiretrovirals come back the next month, and they've put on five kilograms and they are smiling from ear to ear. But for the others, it's heartbreaking. If they had antiretrovirals, they could carry on bringing up their children. They could carry on, and they're not going

to. It is heartbreaking when you know that there is something that can be done, and you actually cannot do it.

Henry Sunpath, Hampton's colleague and the medical director of the AIDS clinic at McCord Hospital, described what was available when a patient had neither an employer nor a family to assist in the purchase of medication.

We offer them very effective and comprehensive treatment with counseling through psychologists, through spiritual counselors and social work support. We assist them [in] making application for disability grants, which are available to patients with advanced disease. We try to get them into our system of comprehensive care and have them come regularly for follow-up and receive treatment for whatever conditions they have. When necessary, we admit them to the acute medical wards, where we treat them for various reversible medical problems. And then we also offer them our palliative medical center, if we find that there is no further cure available for them. We admit them there for just end-of-life care, terminal care, and we afford most of these patients the opportunity to die with dignity, surrounded by their families. Unfortunately, there is an ever-increasing need now for such services. Many of them are dying.

As Jane Hampton noted, the story was very different when antiretrovirals were affordable. Sunpath vividly recounted the story of one patient, a relatively privileged man left impoverished by AIDS, whose family had agreed to pay for his treatment.

He was a 25-year-old man admitted to my medical ward with cryptococcal meningitis. He was extremely ill. He came in knowing his status. And during my talks with him, I encouraged him to come to grips with his diagnosis. He was a computer technologist and was planning to open a business. After two weeks of talk with him and getting his family involved for support, and knowing how much antiretroviral therapy could do, I counseled him, together with them, with his permission, about raising money for antiretroviral drugs. I told his father that if he could only support him for about three or four months, he would be back to work, and he would continue to support himself. His father finally consented.

The patient's CD4 count was 2. It was a great challenge for me to see what was going to happen to this man with such a low CD4. I really wanted to make it work, because he had so many dreams and aspirations; he was trying to begin something great in his life. When he started treatment, we chose a regimen that was most affordable. The problem is that two of the drugs are quite toxic together. Two weeks after starting in, he developed an immune reconstitution syndrome. He developed tuberculosis. We were able to manage that and within that two weeks, we saw him putting on

weight and eating very well. And he was walking around and enjoying a
reasonably good social life at this stage. He also took the courage to tell
his relatives about his state, because he finally realized that "I'm not
actually on death's bed, and I need to tell people. And they need to know
about treatment and living with HIV."

The most remarkable thing about this young man was his determination
to continue despite developing side effects. He had severe peripheral
neuropathy, could not walk for prolonged periods. At night, he had to
lie down in his bed with his feet hanging down. He had to dip them
into cold water constantly. The thing about him is his determination to go
on despite quite severe adverse events. And I always tell him he is my
star patient! And I often tell him, "You need to go out there and speak
to people about what determination is, because part of the success of
it has been your determination."

Not all families could, of course, be counted on to provide the kind of support
Sunpath's patient had received. Aresh Misra, who had initially studied for the
Hindu priesthood and was now in private practice in Durban, recalled one such
patient, who ultimately died of a condition unrelated to AIDS. In this instance it
was an act of generosity by Misra himself that had made treatment possible.

I had a patient who was diagnosed in 1997. He informed his family. They
basically washed their hands of him. A year later, his father brought
him in and said, "I want nothing to do with this guy. He's extremely
ill, don't even give me hope. Just make him comfortable." You can't do
that. You try and treat what is treatable. I examined him and found he
had clinical evidence of TB. I had some samples of antiretrovirals at that
time, a two months' supply. And I put him on that and he did very well. At
that point, his father said, "OK, I will try to get it together and pay for
the medication." They did it for a while. When back at work, he paid
for himself. He had a squabble with his family and became quite sick. I
looked at him and I thought, the family is not going to buy medication.

I put him on until the end. I have a dispensing practice for private patients,
but I never charged him. He actually became part of the practice. He
would come in, and he would help. If there were new patients who wanted
to speak to somebody, I gave them his number. He was comfortable standing up in front of people and telling them, "I have HIV, and I'm not
dead." He became a voluntary counselor, especially for the difficult patients.

The dramatic medical achievements made possible by personal and family
resources or by medical insurance in the private sector, where more than 65 percent of South Africa's doctors served less than 20 percent of its population, were
overshadowed by the state of affairs in the public hospitals and clinics to which

the vast majority of Black South Africans infected with HIV ultimately turned for their care.[2] Most were poor and could rarely count on their families for the kind of financial assistance that antiretroviral treatment required. More often than not, they had no jobs. A deep gulf characterized the nature of the care available to the relatively privileged and those seen in state-run institutions. After completing a clinical consultation with a pregnant woman at King Edward VIII Hospital, Hannah Sebitloane, who had grown up in a rural community in one of apartheid's Black homelands, was forced to face the bitter truth that she could not offer what she knew her patient needed.

> You have gone through the process of discussing everything. You feel
> this particular patient would have definitely benefited from antiretrovirals.
> They would have made a difference in her life. You feel empty. You feel
> maybe it's better if you leave and go to private practice, where you deal with
> a different group of patients, who can better afford them. I thought
> about that. But what about the ones who cannot afford them?

Patients sometimes knew about the new treatments and what they could accomplish. They turned to their doctors, who then had to explain that state hospitals did not make such care available. Bongani Thembela had such encounters at his hospital.

> Fortunately, most of the opportunistic infections we could treat. But
> on their way out, they turn and say, "Doctor, my cousin is taking these
> drugs. Can I get it?" They can see them getting better. Now they want
> to know, and I have to explain that the government policy is this, the pri-
> vate sector is that.

At King Edward VIII's HIV clinic, Sister Gabi Mbanjwa painted a bleak picture of how the cost of treatment affected her patients.

> It's very hard and painful, very hard and painful, because there is no one
> who can afford to buy drugs on a monthly basis for the rest of your life.
> Plus, you have to pay for the viral load test, for the CD4 count test. Even if
> you are having the medical coverage, it is not a joke being a father with
> a family of five. You have to buy this for you, and what about your partner?
> One patient said to me, "I'm the only one that's working. I need to
> prolong my life. But I cannot, because I won't be able to buy the drugs
> for my wife. It's not as if it's me alone."

As he reflected on a patient sent to him by a private practitioner, Paul Nijs, who had worked for the previous 16 years at Edendale Hospital, gave voice to a sense of dismay about the moral foundations of private practice.

A couple of months ago, there was a referral letter from a private doctor, who sent a patient to us. She wrote in her letter, "I refer this patient to you because the patient doesn't have the financial means to be treated by me. So please, can you take over my work?" And then I thought, how must this doctor actually feel, because she is actually unable to help somebody like that—I don't know how many there are, but there must be something like 4 million in South Africa—and she must say, as a doctor, "I cannot help you, because you don't have the money."

Aware of the benefits that could be achieved by treating children with antiretroviral medications, Dalu Ndiweni said simply, "If you have money, you can buy your health. If you have no money, you are damned."

The Burdens of Truth Telling

Given the constraints within which they had to function, caregivers had to decide whether to disclose the benefits of treatment to patients who might not be able to afford antiretrovirals. In this regard, doctors in public hospitals and clinics faced situations not unlike those confronted in the private sector. But the proportion of patients who could conceivably afford antiretroviral therapy was much smaller. Paul Kocheleff described the care with which the staff of his clinic at Grey's Hospital sought to determine whether discussing the possibilities that were available would benefit his patients or cause them suffering.

When we see the patient for the first time, we have a questionnaire. So we have some information about the job they are doing, whether they're working, do they have some income, who is taking care of them financially. We also look at how they are dressed. When the feeling from the information is positive, then I start to ask what the maximum amount of money would be that they could afford per month for treatment. To talk about this medication and to come to the conclusion that it will be totally impossible to buy for a long time will create another stress for these people. And it is not the intention to create it.

Others came to see such caution as unduly paternalistic, depriving patients of the right to know, even if that would leave them despairing or angry. In 2003, Gary Maartens at Groote Schuur explained his decision to shift his approach on this matter.

When antiretroviral therapy first came along in 1996, we weren't really telling our patients, because it wouldn't have helped them a hell of a lot to say, "Look, there is this wonderful treatment, but you are just not going to get it." Then, I took an active policy decision a few years later to say, "Look, this is wrong. We really do need to inform people that this therapy is available in some centers." And if they were rich, they could access it. And when drug companies, at least some of them, started reducing their prices just over two years ago, some of my patients managed to afford to buy their own therapy, either with the help of their families or using their disability pensions.

So it was hard initially even to take that step. It was difficult, because I think it made people unhappy. I hope that we have made some of our patients activists. In fact, I know we have.

For Kogie Naidoo, who had left the care of children and had, by 2000, begun to run the adult HIV clinic at King Edward VIII Hospital, the declining price of drugs and the fact that at least some of her patients might be able to afford treatment meant that failing to tell them about what treatment could do would deprive them of the opportunity to use their resources to obtain the needed money.

Generally, people were not told that antiretrovirals exist, because it wasn't available in the pharmacy of the public hospital. Two years ago, in 2002, a major pharmaceutical firm decided to drop the price of two drugs for triple-therapy patients. They could pay between 400 and 500 rand a month, which was expensive, but not totally out of the range of affordability. Each and every patient who came to the clinic, I felt obliged to tell that therapy exists. I felt it was a way to empower people.

To make treatment more affordable, Naidoo negotiated with private pharmacies to lower their prices for her clinic patients to cost plus a handling fee. She got laboratories to offer their tests at cost. Her efforts paid off, if only very modestly. At the outset, none of her patients was on triple therapy. By 2003, 5 percent were.

There were, however, perils to such an approach. Compelling severely impoverished families to take on the burden of a choice which could mean the difference between life and death was a source of great distress. Tony Moll struggled with this issue, morally troubled by what this decision would mean for his patients and their families.

One of the things I face regularly is the very difficult situation where you have a poor family, one or two working members, and they see their son or their husband following the natural course of the disease. I would like to think, well, maybe they can put it together, and I would like to talk to the family members. And they would say, "Look, we can't afford it at this time, perhaps later on." And then, as time would go on, the patient would get sicker and sicker, and I would approach the subject again. And I would say to the family, "Are you ready?" They will say, "Doctor, we are not ready yet." And then, at a time when the patient is critically ill and imminently dying, the family would then come and say, "OK, doctor, we are ready now." Many times, it's been too late for the patient. That's one of the ethical dilemmas that we face, because family members will try, and feel responsibility. And now the doctor's coming in saying it's a matter of money. You can prolong their family member's life. And they have already had such exhausted resources or poor resources that they blame themselves if they don't manage to do it. And that's [an] incredibly difficult thing to talk to families about. I just continue to grapple with it, and I can say it's something not resolved in my own thoughts. In my own mind, it's an ongoing dilemma.

When, after difficulty, the family could amass enough money to begin treatment, it could, as Tony Moll noted, sometimes be too late. Dalu Ndiweni remembered a mother in 2004 who had agreed to pay for antiretrovirals because she believed that when her own resources were exhausted the government might, at long last, make treatment available. His first contact with this woman's child, who suffered from severe diarrhea and other opportunistic complications, had occurred sometime earlier.

Toward the end, the mother said, "Oh, now I've got a little bit of money. I think I want to start antiretrovirals." At that moment, the child's albumin was low. She had developed malnutrition, that we get in small children, almost a multiple vitamin deficiency, because of ongoing diarrhea. We had done a CD4 count; it was very low. The viral load was very high. And she said, "I want to try. Give her antiretrovirals." And I said, "How long are you going to manage to pay for this?" She replied, "Maybe for four months. I'm hoping in four months the government will have started antiretroviral treatment." So we started. We kept her in hospital for almost a month. The diarrhea stopped eventually. She started eating better. Eventually I said, "Mum, let's try it at home." At home, I think she developed a severe pneumonia. The mother phoned me at three o'clock in the morning and said, "The child has died. She started coughing, and all of a sudden started breathing very fast. And while we're waiting for the ambulance, she stopped breathing."

Beggars Can't Be Choosers

In desperation, some doctors would call upon every resource, their own powers of persuasion, their professional connections, only to confront their own limits. Having told a 25-year-old patient with a CD4 count of 11 and severe opportunistic infections about what treatment she could offer, Farida Amod, an infectious disease specialist at King Edward VIII, hoped that she could make such care available. "I spoke to the mother, I spoke to the aunt, I spoke to the granny," all of whom appeared unable to pay. Amod then turned to a clinic that had funded a number of treatment positions. That too failed. For her, this was a cautionary experience.

> As I built myself up, built my expectations up, I also built her expectations up. At the end, it was tragic, because they couldn't come up
> with the money, and each time she felt that she was going to access
> treatment from somewhere or other. It didn't happen.

Faced with so many dying patients, and the fact that almost none of them could afford the treatment regimens considered appropriate, doctors sometimes took recourse in second-best approaches. Even though a combination of three drugs had become the internationally recognized standard of care, and the use of two antiretroviral drugs in combination was viewed as ultimately ineffective, some saw compromise as both morally and clinically acceptable.

Both highly skilled and imaginative, Leon Levin had established and directed the Pediatric Discussion Group of the Southern African HIV Clinicians Society. He also worked to overcome the nihilism that surrounded the care of children and sought to make dual therapy available in the mid-1990s, just as the international revolution in therapeutics was taking hold. To make the treatment more affordable, he arranged for a chemist to split the capsules of one antiretroviral drug into two. This made possible a 50 percent reduction in price. He then provided the medication to children at cost.

> We got the drugs down to a reasonable price. It was still beyond the reach
> of a lot of people. But at that stage, we were able to offer dual therapy,
> which was reasonably good, at a cheaper price than had they bought
> the medication at a pharmacy.

From her clinical experience in Great Britain in the mid-1990s, Caroline Armstrong, at Grey's Hospital, knew how powerful triple-drug cocktails could be. She nevertheless chose to offer two-drug treatment to those of her patients who could afford it.

> In 2001, the price of two antiretrovirals came down, and now suddenly we
> had a dual-therapy combination we could use, and we were very excited
> about that. We put a lot of patients on dual therapy, even though we knew
> that dual therapy wasn't the way to go. And some people did very well
> on that. But then we started to see side effects, particularly peripheral
> neuropathies. We had four deaths, which was enough to scare us. But what
> do you do? You've got people who have got the choice of that or nothing.

Others sought to make triple-combination therapy affordable by using drugs that had become cheaper because they were no longer being used in wealthy nations. As one doctor observed:

> The impression one gets is that the drugs some patients get are so cheap because they are having difficulty peddling them in other parts of the world because of their toxicity. And that's why they are getting rid of them here. They're going to help quite a few people, even if they do undeniable harm to a select few. But, I suppose, beggars can't be choosers.

There were, however, circumstances in which doctors could prescribe triple-combination therapy using drugs about which there were no such concerns. The experience was transformative. For Eula Mothibi, a visit to her family in Kimberley, the provincial capital of the Northern Cape Province, 600 miles from the Cape Town hospital where she worked, provided her an opportunity to treat a patient with antiretrovirals. Her mother had alerted her to the fact that a relative was very sick.

> I looked at her and I knew. She was pale as a sheet. I touched her. She was hot! I said to her, "You're coming to Cape Town." I took her in my car, which was probably a stupid thing. And I drove all the way from Kimberly, 1,000 kilometers. She was sick. She could have died on the way there. I knew that if I got her to Cape Town, there was a chance that she would live. I got her to the hospital, and they treated her. She was septicemic at the time. She had a CD4 count of 4. I started her on treatment and looked after her at home for a month and a half. She started getting better. She's still alive. Now, she's an HIV counselor.

Kogie Naidoo had a similar experience, which allowed her to regain her sense of agency as a physician, which she had begun to see wane. As she had wanted to empower her patients by informing them about antiretroviral treatment, she herself felt newly enabled.

> I had a patient with severe oral thrush, reactivating TB, and cryptococcal meningitis. He came to the clinic with the CD4 count of about 80. He was extremely wasted. So he came to me and said, "Doctor, I know that this is what's wrong with me, but I don't want to die. My family and I want to do whatever is possible to live." I explained to him about the antiretroviral options and asked him about funding. He was on medical aid.
>
> The first six to eight weeks, he felt wonderful. He was phoning me and thanking me and couldn't believe it. This was a miracle. He had gained 20 kilograms. He was really doing well and was ready to go back to work. Four months into the antiretroviral treatment, he developed reactivation

TB. I had never experienced immune reactivation syndrome. I didn't even know what it was all about. All I knew was this was supposed to be my success story. And here is this guy getting sick. I couldn't understand, and of course I had to go back and read. Eventually, I got him on TB treatment and continued his drugs. He's doing amazingly well. He's an able, productive person. He can support his four kids. And he didn't expect to live.

It was exciting for me. It was scary at the same time, because I was giving him drugs that I was not so familiar with or comfortable with. It was like being on the edge. I felt I was turning the face of this epidemic. If there are some people that I can reach, then I'm going to go ahead and reach them. I feel the need to tell everybody about this and, in so doing, try and help as many people as I can.

But experiences like those of Mothibi and Naidoo, gratifying as they were, only served to place into bold relief the unmet needs of patients for whom the cost of medications were beyond reach.

Inequalities

Inequalities in the care of AIDS patients were embedded in a broader pattern of social inequities in post-apartheid South Africa. The profound differences between private sector medicine and the public sector health care system were obvious to all and were a stark reminder that social class divisions had been carried into a multiracial democracy. There were many reasons that doctors concerned about AIDS chose to care for the relatively narrow stratum who could afford private sector medicine. The ability to earn far more money was obviously a central factor. But there were other reasons as well: frustration with the limits of what they could do for their patients under the prevailing economic and political constraints that defined public medicine; conditions of work that were often exhausting and demoralizing; a belief that the kind of doctor-patient relationship they saw as essential to good medical care was only possible in private practices and hospitals.

Dissatisfied with her isolation in the private practice that she established in 2001, Pinky Ngcakani, nevertheless, recalled her need to leave King Edward VIII Hospital.

Why do they have to die so young? Why do they have to die so painfully? It is traumatic—which is part of my reason for leaving King Edward Hospital. I knew there was no hope in treating those patients. I knew that there was medication out there and our hands were tied. I could never live with myself, knowing that there was medication available and not do anything when there is something I could do better than what I was doing. So

I decided, let me come to private practice, because at least there, there was hope, in the sense that I could provide antiretrovirals.

For Lucky Ndokweni, it was the sheer exhaustion of working in an understaffed public hospital with an unresponsive administration that set the stage for his departure for the private office in Durban where he still worked six days a week.

It was 1995 or 1996 when I was very cross with management, and I told them that I need someone to help me. I cannot run at once the pediatric ward, female ward, and I have to run the operating theaters late, have to do referrals to tertiary hospitals. So that everything rested on me. You were expected to be on call in casualty. It was quite hectic.

But he also felt that private practice afforded him the opportunity to give patients the kind of attention he believed they deserved.

Patients want a relationship with the doctor. They want to sit down and relate to the doctor, not just come in and you say, "There is the medication, go." With HIV patients, you need to educate people about prevention. "You have to use condoms. You cannot conduct your sexual activities recklessly. You still need to use protection."

Aresh Misra, too, starkly contrasted the quality of care that he could provide to his patients as a private practitioner with what he had seen in public settings. His understanding of the ethics of medicine and the demands of the competitive market for patients dictated his choices.

What I found different about the state sector and private sector is the rapport that doctors have with their patients. It was very offhand in the public sector, whereas in the private sector, you have to be a lot more involved, a lot more caring. And you have to give a lot more time to the patients. In the state sector, for doctors, it is just their job. It's a big problem. They get frustrated because they are seeing huge numbers of patients.

In his 12 hour-a-day practice, he strove for more.

You get to know patients. They become friends, and you go to their homes. You have a cup of tea with them, time allowing, and I like practicing medicine that way. I think one of the things that has been extremely successful in growing my practice is my availability to the patient at any time. They have my e-mail address. They have my home number and my cell phone number.

Those who rejected the lure of private practice did not dispute the characterization of the state health care system as radically limiting. But for them, there was no alternative that was morally acceptable. For Kogie Naidoo, it was her experience growing up under the apartheid-imposed separation of the Indian community that was central. "I was very much in touch with people who had no means of accessing private health care. I felt that I needed to serve the wider community as opposed to a small group that could afford it." Farida Amod, whose entire professional life had been in a public hospital, felt that to turn to the private sector, which sometimes beckoned, would be tantamount to desertion.

> In the public sector, I have the opportunity to provide service to people who ordinarily would not have been able to access my skills. One of the things that has impacted most on me is that, in effect, if I had to leave and go into the private sector, many of my patients who have come to depend on me now would not be able to afford my skills. Whenever I get fed up or frustrated, I think, "But who are they going to see?" I'm sure that there are other physicians who can take care of them, but I just somehow feel that they may not have those interpretive skills I've acquired in laboratory.

The inequalities these doctors saw within South African health care seemed to mock the promise of greater equality in the post-apartheid era. Speaking from his office in a private hospital, David Spencer was blunt in his assessment of how the world of privilege had survived the end of racist rule.

> This is a two-tiered system. It's always been. And the reality is, 1994 did not bring a new dispensation in that sense. This is a private hospital. The wealthy, including politicians, come to see me here. For those who manage the health of the nation, it appears acceptable for the indigent to go to government hospitals where you stand in queues or sit for hours and don't get attended to. When those who manage the health of the nation are ill, they come to me and say, "Sort me out. Put me in one of your wards here and look after me."

In Cape Town's premier public hospital, Groote Schuur, Gary Maartens portrayed a troubling situation in South Africa that he saw as inevitable, yet undesirable.

> It's probably like the gulf between medicine in the United States and medicine in a Latin American country. It's a very big gulf, indeed. Virtually anything that you can get in the States, you can get in the private sector, although quite a lot of private medical aid schemes are not able to afford all levels of care. In the public sector, there is a huge staffing

shortfall of doctors, especially in rural areas. There are a lot of inexperienced doctors. They have tried to counter that by having community
service medical officers who go out to rural hospitals. But they are very
inexperienced. They are a year or two out of internship. They generally
run the show, often with private part-time specialists who, in fact, give very
little of their time to the hospitals. There are huge numbers of therapies
that are just unavailable for the vast majority of public sector patients. I
would like to see a health care system that is more equitable. But in
any poor country, you always get a small, wealthy elite, with a giant
gulf between them and the masses, who don't have much. That is a reality of developing countries. It is just a fact. I would like it to be less
obvious.

Without challenging the broader patterns of social inequality, James Muller,
whose administrative duties in Pietermaritzburg's public hospitals had deepened
his understanding, stressed that for him the health care gulf described by Maartens
raised more profound questions about equity in the new South Africa.

If you are a rich man, you get a Mercedes-Benz. If you are a poor man, you
walk; you go and buy a pair of shoes. It doesn't really make that much
of a difference. But if you're a rich man, and you've got a hell of a pain in
your hip, you can get it fixed. But if you are a poor man, and you have
a hell of a pain in your hip, you can't get it fixed. That's not fair.

The differences within South Africa mirrored the chasm between South
Africa—a middle-income country more fortunate than the poorest countries in
Africa—and the industrialized world, where the management of AIDS had un-
dergone a radical transformation since the mid-1990s, where the birth of children
with HIV infection had all but disappeared because of antiretroviral prophylaxis,
where hospital wards were no longer filled with young men and women afflicted by
opportunistic infections, and where death was no longer an immediate expectation
following the diagnosis of HIV infection.
    When, in 1994, Haroon Saloojee read a report of the clinical trial in the United
States which demonstrated that, with AZT, maternal-fetal transmission of HIV
could be reduced radically—by two-thirds—he was immediately struck by how the
cost of that relatively complex intervention would make it inaccessible in South
Africa, where the burden of pediatric AIDS would certainly be greater than in
America.

I remember reading about those results. I think the key figure that stuck
in my mind was the reduction from 24 percent transmission to 8 percent.
I remember that figure clearly. It struck me that there is something you
can really do. My response was twofold: great excitement, because I was

saying, "This is great." And fairly quickly, there was the realization that this was not something we were going to do soon. It was purely a cost issue. It's not going to be affordable.

Half a decade later, when antiretroviral treatment of children with HIV infection had become a standard in wealthy nations, an American lecturer came to Cape Town to describe the new therapeutic prospects. Paul Roux, who through his research and dogged efforts to raise private funds had been able to place children on antiretroviral therapy, recalled his colleagues' absolute disbelief.

An American pediatrician gave a fantastic talk at the University of Stellenbosch. I remember her saying, when she was asked how long the benefit of antiretrovirals last, "I tell the parents that your child will probably survive to see his or her child graduate from college." I remember that phrase. At the end of that talk, every single pediatrician that asked a question asked something like, "Surely, the side effects are dreadful"; "Surely, adherence is impossible"; "Surely, resistance in children happens much more quickly than in adults"; "Surely, the kids hate the taste." I can only interpret these questions as evidence of intense guilt that we didn't have access to the drugs and that there had to be a good reason why we weren't using them.

Those who had worked in or visited countries where a therapeutic transformation had begun in the mid-1990s, or when it was well under way later in the decade, could not help but be struck by the differences. After training in the United States, one physician said, "Coming back in 1996 was like coming to the land of the lotus eaters. Having been exposed to what was going on in America on every level and seen success, it was startling to come back home. There was literally nothing going on, absolutely nothing." Eula Mothibi, another doctor, had worked in Ireland.

It hit me in the face when I came back in 1996. Being able to do nothing in terms of treatment but making patients comfortable. At that time, we didn't even have fluconazole to treat meningitis. So, the only thing we could treat was TB and pneumonia. And if it was bad, and there wasn't anything else, we gave them morphine, Valium, and let the patient pass away quietly. We had Bactrim. It was just not being used for prophylaxis against PCP at the time.

In an epiphanous trip to New York City, where she saw that poor HIV positive children could be as boisterous and healthy as kids used to be in her clinics, Tammy Meyers of Baragwanath Hospital in Johannesburg was struck by what she felt were disturbing global inequities.

I went to Harlem Hospital a few times, and that was for me one of the big, life-changing experiences. Here were these kids in the pediatric AIDS clinic who were in treatment, bouncing into the clinic like any well kid. Comparing that to what we were doing at home was astounding. And that was when I started thinking, We've got to be able to do something about antiretrovirals. Why should these kids have access to this treatment that can save their lives, and we see kids at home that just die?

For infectious disease specialist Farida Amod, who also had visited Harlem Hospital, the contrast with South Africa was both striking and painful. She recalled sitting in on a group of patients infected as the result of intravenous drug use.

They talked about their HIV infection, and they all had these little cards. One guy showed me the card, and it had his CD4, his viral load, the date, and what treatment he was on. I saw that in 1992, he had a CD4 count of 72 and a viral load somewhere in the thousands. And now, eight or nine years later, his CD4 was 600, and his viral load was undetectable. I was so upset. I found it hard that people in America could have it and my patients in South Africa couldn't, just by virtue of the fact that they were South Africans and these were Americans. I just felt we have so many needier patients, patients with children, patients who are working but still cannot afford treatment, and they are not given the opportunity of showing me a card 10 years later. I think that got to me. You need to see people living for a long time to realize that it doesn't have to be this way.

Some reacted to the glaring global disparities by placing them in the broad context of how it was necessary to think about health care in poor countries over the long haul. Paul Nijs thought back to his medical training in Belgium in the early 1970s.

At the School of Tropical Medicine in Antwerp, I remember one professor told us, "The medicine you have learned at university is a medicine that only will reach 20 percent of the world's population. For 80 percent of the world's population, this medicine does not exist. Or they don't have access to it." From that young age, I actually wanted to concentrate on health care that goes to those 80 percent. The fact that antiretrovirals were being used in the First World, that was OK for me in the beginning. It was obviously not an option for us.

Others, especially in the period after 2000, believed that it was necessary to press for change, without illusions about what South Africans could afford to do. In 2003, Gary Maartens, an executive member of the HIV Clinicians Society, said:

> With triple therapy, we could be doing more and should be doing more.
> Hopefully, we will in the near future. But it is unrealistic for us to try
> to mimic what is done in Europe and America. It's ridiculous. We do not
> have the financial resources to do that. We need to do things that are
> more appropriate for our economic situation.

For many others, their ranks swollen by an emerging movement of treatment activists appalled by the absence of effective treatment for AIDS, the gap between what was possible in Europe and America as compared to countries like South Africa made clear the fundamental unfairness of the global distribution of wealth. For them, the response was a rising tide of anger. A senior Black doctor, who had suffered the indignities of the apartheid regime and the inequities of the public hospitals, gave voice to this changing mood.

> Personally, I've had to take a philosophical view. What AIDS is doing is
> exposing the weaknesses in how the human race is organized. It was created
> with haves and have-nots. So what we are seeing now is part of the big-
> ger picture. This is not just with AIDS. So it makes me angry some-
> times. Sometimes, it makes me hate.

Politics Takes Command

Even if the most glaring differences between what was available in the richest countries and in South Africa could not be eliminated, it was possible to think of the prospect of reducing the inequities within South Africa. Only a decision on the part of the government to provide access to antiretrovirals for the prevention of mother-to-child transmission of HIV or for treatment would have put an end to rationing by ability to pay. Given the cost of the medications, it was an option that many believed was beyond the state's fiscal capacity. Inevitably, questions arose about why drugs were so costly. Pharmaceutical firms became the objects of scathing analyses. Critics began to challenge the global system of patents, which served to protect corporate investments and profits.[3]

Although claims about the cost of treatment would remain a leitmotif of government pronouncements in the late 1990s and the first years of the twenty-first century, an unexpected and almost inexplicable turn in official outlook would place the government of Thabo Mbeki, Nelson Mandela's successor as president, on a collision course with almost all physicians, scientists, AIDS activists, and the ANC's own political allies. The state itself would emerge as the most persistent obstacle to the provision of antiretrovirals to South Africans suffering from AIDS.

The government's antagonism extended beyond the role of antiretrovirals as therapy to their potential use as a prophylaxis against mother-to-child transmission of HIV. Furthermore, in 1999, the Minister of Health announced that she would not permit the provision of AZT to women who had been raped, an intervention that could, it was believed, based on the experience of wealthy nations, prevent infection, as did the prophylactic treatment of health care workers who had suffered needle stick injuries. Research was necessary, said the minister, to establish both efficacy and safety. But the research she demanded—involving a control group that would remain untreated—was viewed by many as simply unethical.[4]

Only gradually did it become clear that Thabo Mbeki was shaping the responses of his health minister. Toward the end of 1999, he told a meeting of provincial health officials that he thought AZT might be harmful to those for whom it was prescribed.[5] The annual report of the African National Congress that year stated that AZT would not be made available because of remaining questions about safety and efficacy.[6]

In the spring of 2000, according to South Africa's prominent newspaper the *Mail and Guardian*, Mbeki contacted an American scientist who had rejected the idea that HIV was the cause of AIDS and sought his advice on how he might best evaluate the evidence on the matter. Soon thereafter, he wrote that proponents of antiretrovirals had sacrificed their intellectual integrity by becoming salespersons for Glaxo-Wellcome, the manufacturer of AZT. This was a theme to which he and other ANC officials would often return. Speaking to his political base, the caucus of ANC parliamentary members, he said:

> If one agreed that HIV caused AIDS, it followed that the condition had
> to be treated by drugs. And those drugs were produced by the Western drug
> companies. The drug companies therefore needed HIV to cause AIDS.
> So they promoted the thesis that HIV caused AIDS.[7]

On May 4, 2000, Mbeki appointed an international presidential panel composed equally of proponents and opponents of the scientific claim that HIV was the viral cause of AIDS, charging it with the responsibility of reporting back their findings.[8] Physicians and scientists within South Africa and abroad looked on in dismay as this process unfolded, just as final preparations were being made for the biennial international gathering of AIDS specialists that was to take place in Durban in July 2000. When the world gathering occurred, in the presence of a huge press corps, the views of the South African government were repeatedly pilloried. Jerry Coovadia, professor of pediatrics at Durban's Nelson R. Mandela School of Medicine and chair of the conference, recalled:

> On the opening day of the conference, we had a magnificent speech by
> Judge Edwin Cameron, a gay man living with AIDS, which just lambasted
> the government. The first scientific speech was by David Ho, the inter-

nationally recognized authority, who had a picture of the HIV virus on the screen behind him, and he said, "This is the HIV virus. And I want to tell you that it causes AIDS." He got a standing ovation. So, from day one, the government was under attack.

As chair of the conference, Coovadia was pressed at a meeting attended by Health Minister Manto Tshabalala-Msimang and several provincial health ministers to provide her with the opportunity to address the conference so that the South African government might defend itself. He demurred, arguing that he did not have the authority to alter a program agreed to by a scientific advisory panel. Minister Tshabalala-Msimang, he recalled, told him that he was "disloyal." And then one of the assembled officials said to him, "Tomorrow, your international friends will be gone, and then there will be you and then there will be me. And we will then see."

Coovadia found these words painful and shattering. To a man who had been active in the anti-apartheid struggle, and for whom the bombing of his home by the South African police was a defining experience, to be spoken to in such a manner was almost beyond comprehension. During the most brutal days of apartheid, he said, "I never bowed down to a policeman or a Boer, never compromised my integrity. I fought, no matter how scared I was. But this thing really rocked me."

So furious did the increasingly embattled official government position become that, in the northern province of Mpumalanga, the provincial health minister sought to evict a rape crisis center operated by a nongovernmental organization from a public hospital, because it was prescribing antiretrovirals to its clients, providing them free of charge.[9] An officially inspired petition signed by some hospital workers revealed the vitriolic tone of the increasingly common assaults on those who opposed government policy. The petition charged the clinic with attempting to "drug our people to death.... We cannot defy our President Thabo Mbeki and his call against AZT."[10] Others invoked the image of biological warfare against Black people.[11]

For Mbeki and his political allies, the belief that a sexually transmitted virus was the cause of AIDS ignored the ways in which poverty and malnutrition were at the root of the illnesses that afflicted Black people. It was deeply offensive. It was nothing less than a new expression of the racism that had always sought to demean and subjugate Black Africans. In a speech given in the fall of 2001, the president said:

> Others who consider themselves to be our leaders take to the streets
> carrying their placards to demand that, because we are germ carri-
> ers and human beings of a lower order that cannot subject their pas-
> sion to reason, we must perforce adopt strange opinions to save
> a depraved and diseased people from perishing from a self-inflicted
> disease.[12]

Nothing more dramatically illustrates the scope of the antagonism toward the doctors and scientists who, with increasing despair, believed their government to be in the thrall of a madness with life-and-death implications for their patients, than the publication in 2002 of *Castro Hlongwane, Caravans, Cats, Geese, Foot and Mouth and Statistics.*[13] A biting ideological diatribe against antiretroviral therapy and the clinicians who championed such care, the authorship was traced to the office of the president.[14] Discussed by the national executive committee of the ANC and distributed to its branches, *Castro* reprised the assertions that those who criticized the government's position were guilty of betrayal, craven capitulation to foreign influence, and racism.

> Stridently and openly, the omnipotent apparatus disapproves of our ef-
> fort seriously to deal with the serious challenge of our . . . health, pov-
> erty and underdevelopment. . . . All of us are obliged to chant that
> HIV = AIDS = Death! We are obliged to abide by the faith, and no other,
> that our immune systems are being destroyed solely and exclusively by
> the HI Virus. We must repeat the catechism that sickness and death among
> us are primarily caused by heterosexually transmitted HI Virus. Then
> our government must ensure that it makes antiretroviral drugs available
> throughout our public health system.[15]

The document went on to hold individual doctors and scientists culpable for those who died in the course of antiretroviral research.

> Pregnant women have died because they were subjected to these "safe,
> effective and tolerable alternatives"! Reportedly one of them is a Black
> woman, on whom Glenda Gray experimented with toxic drugs at
> Chris Hani Baragwanath Hospital. . . . Since Glenda Gray must be held
> accountable, how has this been expressed? Since Chris Hani Baragwanath
> Hospital must be held accountable, how has this been expressed?[16]

For Glenda Gray, who viewed her lifelong commitment to the struggle of those who had been oppressed by the apartheid regime as self-defining, to be denounced in so bitter and threatening a manner was deeply disturbing. Like Jerry Coovadia, she had begun to understand that the political bonds forged in the years of opposition to apartheid had little to do with how the government would treat those who now confronted it on AIDS.

> They accused me of being a murderer of Black pregnant women. That
> for me was scary, because it was like I had come around the whole circle
> from having this feeling under apartheid, and now, having this feeling
> under the new dispensation. Have things changed?

By 2003, when the minister of health would assert that olive oil, garlic, and African potato might be more effective in treating AIDS than antiretrovirals,[17] and when the minister of finance was reported to have said that spending money on antiretrovirals was like spending money on voodoo medicine,[18] a number of physicians began to denounce the government in language that would have been unthinkable a few years earlier, following the end of apartheid. Speaking about President Mbeki's history of resistance to providing effective drug treatment to people with AIDS, Haroon Saloojee, a neonatologist, said in 2003:

> This is the antithesis of everything that the struggle was about. We were fighting for democracy, for people's rights. We have allowed our own government, a democratic government, to basically allow 50,000 babies to die each year. I think history will view the actions of this government, as regards HIV/AIDS, very seriously. I am still a supporter of the ANC, but this is genocide.

James McIntyre, Saloojee's colleague at Baragwanath Hospital, who with Glenda Gray received the prestigious Nelson Mandela Award for Health and Human Rights in 2002, drew the only possible conclusion, given the invocation of genocide. He boldly asserted, "They are going to have to go on trial. They are guilty of human rights atrocities, from Mbeki, down to the national Department of Health. We can intervene, and all that is happening is obstruction left, right, and center."

Black doctors and nurses felt similar outrage. But it was not as easy for them to invoke the language of trials and genocide against the governing ANC, which had led the struggle against apartheid. Clarence Mini, whose grandmother had been arrested as an ANC activist in the 1960s and who had been recruited into the ANC in 1976, said that the party was "like a home." There was no possibility of struggling for a change in AIDS policy outside of the ANC.

Nevertheless, the stage had been set for a titanic struggle in South Africa, one that would shatter the hopes and the illusions about how liberation movements, turned into governing parties, would act when faced with a crisis of legitimacy. AIDS was, it was now clear, not simply a challenge to health; it struck at the very social fabric of South Africa. In its response, the ANC government would expose to many AIDS caregivers elements of rigidity and authoritarianism that would tarnish the currency it had acquired as the successor to one of the late twentieth century's most moving struggles for freedom and human dignity.

5

Defiance

Creating Islands of Treatment

Despite the government's intransigence regarding antiretroviral treatment, islands of access to such care for those who could not otherwise afford it began to materialize late in the 1990s. Clinical investigators were able to capitalize on the interests of pharmaceutical firms in conducting research in South Africa. International humanitarian relief organizations, appalled by the scale of the evolving epidemic, sought to underwrite limited treatment efforts. And within the corporate sector, some of South Africa's largest firms extended medical coverage to include antiretroviral therapy (ART), either through health insurance or directly through company clinics.[1] Those who pressed for such innovations believed that by demonstrating the efficacy of treatment for people with AIDS, they would not only meet the clinical needs of patients but provide a powerful antidote to the secrecy and stigmatization that had so defined the social response to AIDS.

For those doctors and nurses whose perspective was informed by a commitment to changing policy, such innovative efforts provided the occasion for witnessing the extraordinary power of ART to restore desperately sick, sometimes dying, patients to health, work, and their families. These experiences only served to reinforce their commitment to fundamentally changing the government's posture on AIDS. To those whose work was informed by a clinical perspective, within which the needs of their own patients provided the motivating force for circumventing governmental restrictions, the ability to reach out to a limited number only served to underscore the inequity of piecemeal responses to an epidemic of socially catastrophic proportions.

Research as Treatment

Even before the South African government began its ideological campaign against antiretroviral drugs, clinicians in the public sector, who wanted to give their patients some opportunity to benefit from treatments available to AIDS patients in wealthy nations, sought to broaden the prospects of access through drug trials and other research undertakings. For pharmaceutical firms, in turn, South Africa provided an ideal setting. As Gary Maartens at Groote Schuur Hospital in Cape Town observed:

> We had tons and tons of patients who had never smelled antiretrovirals, so that we could get the numbers up very fast. We are a cheap place to do research. Clinicians are cheap here. Nurses are cheap here. Lab investigations are cheap here. Such trials benefited both patients and doctors. On the plus side, they enabled us to use the drugs on public sector patients; we treated several hundred. It was great for our patients to have the disease turned around instead of going downhill all the time.

Maartens also noted that money paid by pharmaceutical firms helped to fund his other research operations. Characterizing the situation, he said it was "win-win. Everybody was happy."

Trial participants were at the same time patients. As researchers, physicians could, at last, become effective clinicians. Robin Wood, at the time working at Cape Town's Somerset Hospital, which had pioneered the treatment of gay men with AIDS in the 1980s, was among the first to take this route.

> It was only in 1995 and 1996 when we started performing clinical trials, and the reason for that was that we recognized that this was a way of getting access to therapy in a medical system that wouldn't pay for monitoring or for drugs.

Wood's efforts were facilitated by a cooperative hospital administration. But even in the years before Thabo Mbeki launched his assault on the treatment establishment, Wood felt it necessary to be circumspect, to be "fairly quiet about it to begin with." It was based on that work that he and his colleagues realized that extending their efforts would necessitate going beyond hospital-based drug trials. Community-based efforts—dubbed "operational research"—would permit them to gain experience in the provision of care to larger numbers without openly contravening the government's antipathy to ART. By 2004, he had been able to offer treatment to 600 patients.

For Tammy Meyers at Baragwanath, it had been the experience of seeing the vitality of treated children with AIDS at New York's Harlem Hospital that had driven her to enter the world of international clinical trials.

> Why should these kids have access to this treatment that can save their lives, and we see at home kids that just die? If we had clinical trials, we would be able to at least offer it to some kids. I thought that was the way to

go. It was just not possible to provide antiretroviral treatment to people cared for in the public service, who are mostly indigent. In 2000, the U.S.-based Pediatric AIDS Clinical Trial Group started putting out applications. We put in an application and actually got awarded the grant, and that gave us extra funding.

She then teamed up with Harlem pediatricians for a successful application to the U.S. National Institutes of Health. Hers was a small trial involving only 30 children.

As knowledge of such clinical trials began to spread, some HIV patients began to assert that they had a right to be research subjects. In South Africa, as had been the case in the United States a decade earlier, this upended the conventional view that clinical research posed a potential burden against which vulnerable individuals needed protection. Glenda Gray, whose patients came from Soweto, recalled:

A woman came to me and said, "How come if you are white and gay and live in Johannesburg, you can get into a treatment trial? How come you don't get us into these treatment trials?" So in 1996, we started approaching drug companies, and at first no one would touch them because they were Black women. They were illiterate. They lived in shacks. They were not going to take their medicine. They were going to fall out of studies. So nobody would give it to us.

Luckily, a former classmate was the medical director of the South African division of a major international pharmaceutical firm. Gray approached her about the possibility of enrolling Black women. Ultimately she was told, "We will cut you some slack and give you one study."

For doctors working in the public sector, who had read and heard about what antiretroviral treatment could do but who had no firsthand experience of just how dramatic a clinical impact these drugs could have, the first patients brought into a trial could provide memorable moments. It was in 2003 that Tony Moll, whose rural hospital had provided a model of AIDS care with everything but antiretrovirals, started his first participants in a project jointly undertaken with the veteran American AIDS clinician Gerald Friedland of Yale University.[2]

We had a small group of five patients that we started together. Three of them had very low CD4 counts, under 50. I knew that two of them would not survive another few months without antiretroviral therapy. One girl had a CD4 count of 10; she was the mother of a little child at home. She actually had Kaposi's sarcoma already in her mouth and some other places on her body. The other lady was a mother of two young boys, already school-going; her CD4 count was 38, and she was thin and wasted. We took photographs that day when they started their medication.

Two weeks later, they came back, and, boy, they had moans and groans. It was vomiting. It was diarrhea. It was this and that. And we sat around in a group. Everybody shared what they were feeling, what they were experiencing. We encouraged them. For us, it was kind of embarking on something new for the patients. From their side, it was embarking on something new. It was kind of bad, hearing all the problems and having to reassure them, not being quite sure, you see! One girl developed a skin rash. It wasn't that bad, but just to be sure, we admitted her. At the end of the first month, two of the patients had lost weight and had got[ten] worse. I telephoned Dr. Friedland, and he said, "Don't worry. Just carry on. It's reconstitution syndrome. Just keep on. It's going to sort itself out." At the end of two months, they had more or less stabilized, and it was in the third month that they all took an amazing leap forward. One guy gained six kilograms; the others gained two, three, and four. That was the very first time that with our own eyes, under our own hands, with our own experience, we saw the turnaround take place. Two patients were brought back from the very brink of death.

Given the ongoing hostility of the minister of health to the use of antiretrovirals and persistent official suggestions that such drugs would be deleterious to the sick, even poisonous, Moll was especially alert to the impact of this new effort on his staff.

The whole staff was watching in the wings now. What's going to happen? And does this stuff really work? It took three months, I must say, of being ambivalent. But when those weights came back and the patients started looking good and feeling good and we'd gone past those initial side effects, it was very reassuring to the staff. That's when they started really believing in antiretrovirals. They trusted me, but they had to see with their own eyes what would actually happen.

But whatever they could mean for patients who were selected for trials that guaranteed access to antiretroviral treatment, such efforts, by definition, had to exclude many more than could be offered medication. And, thus, rationing potentially life-saving care characterized the world of trials as it did the world of clinical care more generally. With the number of participants limited, doctors and the nurses who worked at their sides had to engage in a process of selection. For some, it felt like "playing God." Given the significance of these decisions, Tammy Meyers was "not proud" as she thought back on the approach she had used to choose the children for her first trial.

We had files of the children who attended our clinic and their telephone numbers. It was probably in alphabetical order. We phoned, and whoever we got on the other end of the line was chosen. If they didn't have a phone, we couldn't get hold of them. Sometimes, we did try and send messages off, but it was a rapid enrollment.

Research projects also typically entailed a series of stringent selection criteria. In the township of Guguletu outside of Cape Town, an operational research program was established to circumvent governmental restrictions on the provision of antiretrovirals in public clinics. A team of health workers weighed a complex set of selection guidelines before engaging in what Linda-Gail Bekker called "the Solomon thing." In 2003, the 41-year-old Zimbabwe-born doctor explained that, to be chosen, patients had to live within the district, had to have attended the HIV clinic for six months regularly, and had to regularly come to its meetings. In addition, breaking the isolation imposed by the stigma attached to AIDS, candidates for treatment had to have revealed the fact that they were infected to at least one other person in the community. They also had to agree to have a counselor who would monitor their adherence to treatment. Finally, patients had to be physically able to come to the clinic on their own. This last requirement was not simply a matter of practicality, but was also a way of excluding those who were too debilitated. Some patients, said Bekker, were just too ill to benefit. Efforts on their behalf would distract attention from individuals who might be saved. But there was a second reason for such limitations, one that was intimately connected to the precarious political context within which her clinic operated. Relentless hostility toward antiretroviral treatment by the government, and the confusion such hostility sowed among ordinary men and women, imposed obligations involving institutional survival. "We had to make sure that they were not too sick. Too sick patients have a very high mortality, and that is tough on the program. It feeds the propaganda that drugs are toxic."

Like so many others involved in difficult rationing choices, Bekker believed that it was important that clear rules of selection guide the process. Such rules could prevent favoritism from intruding upon selections that were, she understood, matters of life and death. Nevertheless, she was compelled to acknowledge that the force of an individual personality, of all-too-human emotion, could break through the constraints erected against such impulses.

I had a young woman who had quite severe pulmonary hypertension. She was quite breathless, and the question was, Is this the reason to give her drug to somebody else who will live longer, because she has another illness which might kill her before the HIV does? So we had agreed on every other front: she was treatment ready; she was psychologically sound; she filled all the other criteria. But what about her physical state? And she must have gotten wind that she was hanging in the balance. As I walked into the clinic, she did some star jumps and jumped up and down and moved her arms, and she said, "See, I am fine. I am absolutely fine." There was just no way that I could actually say she mustn't get the drug. I mean, there are just times when somebody's needs and psychology, and the fact that they are human beings, just overwhelms every sense of better judgment. I didn't even examine her. I walked straight out and said, "She has to go into treatment. I can't refuse."

Tony Moll also had to face the challenge of pressures that might mount and threaten the integrity of his trial.

We chose them because they were sick. We had very strict criteria set down by Yale University as to who could get in and who couldn't. What we feared was families or other people actually coming and demanding the medicine, saying, "We've heard that so and so is on medication. We also want it." So in fact those first few patients were given the message, We would like to put everybody on medication, but we don't have it. You guys are the first that we can use it on. Now just be careful with what you say in the community, because we don't want you jumping around and shouting, telling everybody. And I think for the patients that took it, it's been quite a valuable secret that they kept and went home with. In those days, we were very, very clear about not raising expectations and not raising hopes amongst people that we wouldn't be able to meet.

But, as with Linda-Gail Bekker, the rules of inclusion could at times seem unacceptably rigid and cruel, and when that occurred, the rules themselves might have to bend.

Each person participating had to bring a family member who knew and understood their status. They came along and actually went through the training sessions with the patients themselves. There was one study patient whose wife came to us and asked for treatment. It was quite difficult for us to say, "Your husband qualifies, but you don't." We spoke to Dr. Friedland at Yale about this, and he immediately opened the door and said that, if you have a spouse, just put them on the medication as well.

Ironically, clinical trials that had the potential to provide access to treatment to those who would otherwise find medication beyond reach could, at times, serve to underline the social inequalities that so defined treatment opportunities in South Africa. In Pietermaritzburg, Caroline Armstrong described a drug trial at Grey's Hospital that was only open to patients who had failed on a first-line regimen, for which they had been able to pay. Addressing the equity concerns posed by this situation, she said in a matter-of-fact manner, "That's right. It's all down to the money."

Drug trials were also by definition time limited. In a context where the ability to gain access to effective therapy was dependent on such investigations, it was inevitable that questions would surface about what would happen to participants when studies came to an end. Would pharmaceutical firms continue to provide drugs free of charge and, if so, for how long? For those responsible for overseeing the ethics of clinical trials, issues of equity were placed into bold relief. Would excessive demands serve as a disincentive to pharmaceutical firms drawn by the low cost of research in South Africa? And if those costs rose, would trials shift to more favorable settings, depriving the most impoverished of their only hope for access to treatment?

At Groote Schuur Hospital, Paul Roux, who, through research efforts, had been able to place many children on antiretrovirals, noted that he could only guarantee the mothers of those he treated that their sons and daughters would receive treatment for three years. As someone who had studied bioethics and had served on his hospital's institutional review board, he described the situation facing South Africa in the period when the government provided no antiretroviral treatment in stark terms.

> I have heard that in KwaZulu-Natal, for example, a research ethics committee approved a study which would have enabled 40 children to go on antiretrovirals for a guaranteed extra five years poststudy. Which, if you are a beggar, is a good deal. Usually, it's about four and a half years. Anyway, the university approved it, but local government has to approve everything that university does, and they turned it down on the grounds that they wanted lifelong therapy. You can't expect a drug company to do that; that's the sort of thing governments have to do.

At Baragwanath Hospital, Glenda Gray recalled the irony of her encounter with an ethics committee whose concerns about exploitation threatened her patients' well-being.

> The first time we submitted this trial to the ethics committee, they turned it down, because they said the pharmaceutical company promised to give us two years of drugs afterwards, and that wasn't enough. The committee wanted it to be lifelong. We told the women in our support group, and the women said, "No, we want to meet this ethics committee." A meeting was arranged to give the women of Soweto an opportunity to address the academics on the ethics committee. "I'm HIV infected and I am dying," said one woman. "I can be on this trial for two years, and if I do well, I've got another two years' access. That's four years, and you are turning this down, so you are killing me."

Gray wryly observed, "There was this ethics committee of white, middle-aged men who looked at these women and for the first time were confronted with these kinds of issues." The committee yielded. But there remained the issue of how to protect the medically desperate from exploitation.

At Groote Schuur, Gary Maartens, who had been involved in 15 clinical trials dating from the early 1990s and who had described research on antiretrovirals with those who could otherwise not afford it as "win-win," remained deeply ambivalent about his own actions.

> It troubled us from the beginning. It troubled us increasingly as the trials were being conducted. We kept reminding our patients, as it came to the end of the study, look, you know you need to make plans. So we did what we could to help the patients. It did trouble us. Maybe not as much as it should have. But we didn't say no, we said yes. Most of the patients knew from the start that they would get therapy for X years. How would you feel if I said to you, "You can take therapy for two years, or carry on getting nothing?"

Maartens noted that, toward the end of the 1990s, trials increasingly offered extended postinvestigation treatment to those who were responding, including lifelong coverage. But when a trial with less generous provisions presented itself in 2000, he did not turn it down.

> We were intent on the study, where we knew the trial was for one year. And then they got free therapy for two years afterwards. Full stop. We knew that. Our ethics committee knew that. We did it again with open eyes. But in a way, it's a bit like the rationing of the ICU. It was absolutely frightening.

Looking back on his years of involvement with research, he said in 2003, "A lot of good came out of it. I don't feel like it was dirty money. But I don't feel clean and decent about it either."

In some public hospitals, the very effectiveness of placing large numbers of patients into treatment through clinical trials was seen as a rebuke to government policy. At Johannesburg Hospital, Ian Sanne, who headed such investigations, was ultimately forced to move.

> My clinic was initially tolerated. Eventually, we were having so much influence that the Johannesburg Hospital kicked us out, because we were flying in the face of the national Department of Health that was refusing to have anything to do with antiretroviral therapy. Our results were showing up the minister's and the president's opinion, because we were showing that we could deliver antiretroviral therapy effectively, successfully, safely— and this was counter to what the minister of health was saying. That this was a research undertaking also became very controversial, because the minister of health also targeted antiretroviral therapy research through a very public campaign, calling everybody who participated "guinea pigs."

They were calling us, the researchers, people who were taking advantage of underprivileged Black patients.

But whatever the limits of research as a strategy for opening access to treatment, not all hospitals had the capacity to launch such efforts. Some simply did not have the personnel or resources to make the commitment required by clinical trials. Speaking in 2003, James Muller, who knew intimately the capacity of Pietermaritzburg's three main public hospitals, said, "We have hardly done any research. We have really been snowed under with service burdens, and we have not had the option of doing research." For his patients, too poor to buy their own medication, AIDS care without antiretrovirals was all there was.

The Struggle to Reduce Mother-to-Child Transmission of HIV

Outside the context of research, the struggle to gain access to antiretroviral drugs in the public sector did not begin with the effort to meet the therapeutic needs of those who were infected with HIV but rather with the goal of preventing transmission of the virus from pregnant women to their babies. In 1994, a research study in the United States had found that the provision of AZT to pregnant women and their newborns reduced the risk of HIV transmission by two-thirds. Despite the cost of the new regimen, there were calls in South Africa as early as 1995 to make the intervention available.[3] Given the toll in human suffering and the cost of treating babies and children with AIDS, some asserted that the preventive regimen met the test of cost-benefit analysis.[4]

Strikingly, opposition to such proposals came from a physician who would emerge as one of the fiercest advocates for mother-to-child prevention efforts and who, as a consequence, would become engaged in a bitter encounter with the government.[5] James McIntyre, who by the mid-1990s had already had extensive experience with the problems presented by AIDS to obstetrical care at Baragwanath Hospital, recalled, "It was obvious that this drug regimen wasn't going to be possible on a wide scale because of cost and implementation issues."

Hovering like a specter over the question of mother-to-child transmission, and with clear implications for the ultimate efficacy of any pharmacological intervention, was the issue of infant breastfeeding. It was clear that HIV could be carried in a mother's milk. Yet breastfeeding was also known to provide infants with great advantages, nutritionally and immunologically. This was especially the case where water supplies themselves posed a threat to newborns. How then was one to balance the risk of HIV transmission against the medical benefits of breast milk? And how were the cultural factors that so defined the centrality of breastfeeding to be considered, given the threat posed by AIDS? Early in the AIDS epidemic, UNICEF had made a determination that infected women in wealthy nations should bottle feed but that women in the Third World should, despite the risks, continue to breastfeed. On this matter, a deep and bitter conflict emerged within South Africa among those who would in other circumstances find themselves allied against the government. Pediatrician Glenda Gray, McIntyre's colleague, believed that the prevailing international standard was unacceptably broad. Within South Africa—in Soweto, for example—there were settings where the water supply would permit the safe use of infant formula, and she believed that the failure to inform women of their options represented a human rights violation. Her encounter, in the mid-1990s, "with the Holy Grail of breastfeeding" made her anathema to some.

> Here I was, this 32-year-old young upstart, saying that women in Africa could safely bottle feed. I was accused of being on the payroll of Nestlé. I was quite naïve. I didn't understand how strong the breastfeeding paternity was. I was a political activist in the country, and I was outraged by these kinds of statements. Jerry Coovadia and I still fight about it. UNICEF kept on asking me who was funding my research. We were not recommending it for all settings. But women who are HIV positive and are poor are entitled to know about the information and to be supported in their decisions.

Commenting on the ways that well-meaning doctors, committed to the welfare of their patients, would go well beyond the provision of information that would permit women to make their own choices, Saul Johnson, like Gray, a pediatrician, recalled that in the 1990s:

> I think on both sides of the debate, we were probably a little bit overzealous and, I think, influenced the women unfairly. I can certainly say that at Baragwanath there was a lot of pressure on the women not to breastfeed, not from us necessarily overtly, but a social norm developed. Women picked that up, and if they saw somebody that appeared to be breastfeeding, waiting for an appointment, there would be lots of talking and chattering. "Oh, you've got to formula feed because that's best for your baby."
>   Then, of course, we got to a point where we had to say, if we believe this, then we have an ethical obligation to try and help these women find the formula. So we had to go and negotiate deals ourselves with the formula companies. And then we would sell it to the women. We subsidized them even more, because we said we'd pay for their transport.

Jerry Coovadia, who viewed the efforts of the infant formula industry as a malevolent force and who had come to believe that consistent breastfeeding, in fact, protected babies from HIV transmission, could not forgive Gray's naiveté, although he understood that she, like he, was a stalwart in the struggle to make the government fund mother-to-child HIV prevention programs. He said,

I must find a solution to the transmission of HIV through breast milk which is applicable to the majority of women. And the overwhelming majority of women are African and they are Indian and there are going to be Chinese tomorrow. These are overwhelmingly poor, so we've got to find a solution for them which is rational, scientific. That's my starting point. The second point is that, unlike some of the others, I've lived through the immense struggle we had for the preservation of breastfeeding, when we were under attack by the large formula-feeding companies, and there was a whole movement throughout the world which fought for breastfeeding. As head of department, I never allowed Nestlé to put a toe into our department. It was an important fight, like our current fight against the larger pharmaceuticals.

You can't just discard breastfeeding; it's a cultural attribute whose benefits go back centuries. So you have got to have a global and historical view. As we are living through this epidemic, what must we do here? The easiest thing in the world is to say, "Let's give formula feeding." It requires no intelligence whatsoever, no imagination whatsoever; to me, that's just too glib.

They talk about the possibilities in Soweto. I have told them a million times, "Soweto is not Africa." Soweto was the jewel in the crown of apartheid. They wanted to show that they were caring for Black people, so when visitors came around, they would show them Soweto and ask them to compare that to the slums in Nairobi.

We have subsidized formula in a country like South Africa. It's a disaster. We now start back to the problems of formula feeding and water and sanitation and diarrhea and pneumonia.

Despite their profound and acrimonious disagreements over breastfeeding, circumstances would compel Gray, McIntyre, and Coovadia to collaborate. Together, they were brought to Geneva by the Joint United Nations Program on AIDS to chart an international research effort that could determine whether a simpler and far shorter course of AZT than what was used in wealthy nations for pregnant women could be effective in reducing mother-to-child transmission of HIV. Were that to be the case, it might then be possible to mount efforts that were affordable in the nations where pediatric AIDS represented a pressing challenge. The multinational UN-organized study would, however, itself become the subject of a bitter international controversy over the conduct of clinical trials.

Conventionally, the ethics of such investigations dictated that the use of placebos could only be justified when there was no extant effective treatment. When effective care was available, controlled trials had to compare proposed interventions against such treatment. But never before had the question of the applicability of such an ethical norm been systematically confronted when the standard of care was unaffordable in poor nations. The emergency posed by AIDS only seemed to

intensify the debate. McIntyre recalled that the issue of trial design had been
discussed in Geneva.

> The discussion was, Should the short course be compared to the more
> expensive complex regimen? And the feeling was that, no, we shouldn't,
> because it wasn't obtainable. It wasn't achievable and wasn't going to be the
> issue. So I'm not saying that there was no consideration of whether [or] not
> to use a placebo, but there was very broad consensus that that was not
> appropriate.

McIntyre, Gray, and Coovadia, who by personal history and current commitment saw themselves as serving the interests of those who had been oppressed
by apartheid, were involved in the conduct of the trial in South Africa. They were
stunned when a bitter denunciation of the effort of which they were a part was
launched by Marcia Angell, the editor of the preeminent *New England Journal of
Medicine*. Invoking the international code of research ethics and the most notorious example of the exploitation of poor research subjects in the United States, she
wrote in September 1997:

> The Declaration of Helsinki requires control groups to receive the "best"
> current treatment, not the [best] local one. The shift in wording between
> "best" and "local" may be slight, but the implications are profound. Ac-
> ceptance of this ethical relativism could result in widespread exploitation of
> vulnerable Third World populations for research programs that could not
> be carried out in the sponsoring country.... It seems as if we have not
> come very far from Tuskegee after all.[6]

It was the comparison to the infamous Tuskegee syphilis trial—in which infected African-American men in Alabama were enrolled, beginning in the 1930s, in
an ongoing investigation which deceptively deprived them of effective treatment
for their disease—that most enraged Coovadia.

> It was a small group of people, in the U.S. primarily, which had exaggerated
> notions of what their responsibilities to humankind were and their arro-
> gance that we were not similarly concerned about the welfare of our own
> people that got to us. It was their arrogance that the Tuskegee example
> applied to us. I was in the wards. I am not only a pediatrician; I just
> happened to also be part of the democratic struggle for freedom in this
> country. So I am not going to listen to somebody sitting in a warm office in
> Boston. In addition to the science, which was a problem, it was just the
> offensiveness of this example of Tuskegee applying to us as if we were
> racially discriminating against Black people. It was just such a horrendously
> awful analogy which offended me.

"We thought," said McIntyre, who with Gray had directed an HIV research unit at Baragwanath since 1991, "we were doing something really good, and we were coming up against this vitriolic attack." To meet this challenge, he and Gray

went back to the women in the trial and the women in the clinic. For four or five weeks in a row, we held town hall meetings with them and discussed the issues that had been raised and offered to stop the study. We actually had somebody in from UNAIDS who came and spoke to them on their own and tried to assess whether they really knew what was happening. They also had discussions with the ethics committee. The thing that stood out for me was the fact that [the patients] were saying, "We understood this and we are not only doing this for us." One woman stood up and said, "No, you must carry on. This is our study, and I know that I might get placebo, but I am not only doing this for me, I am doing it for my sister and for the people out there as well." It was something that I guess I knew. But what was really reinforced was that there was almost a perception that poor people can only have as a reason for taking part in research tradeoffs for their own benefit. And that's not necessarily true. I think it was an important lesson.

The women involved in the trial, Gray recalled, sought assurance that their altruism would not be misappropriated. They told her:

"We will continue with this trial and we will be part of your experiment, but if this trial works, you will have to promise us that you will make these drugs available to every woman in Soweto afterwards. We will go on placebo for that." And then I promised that, if the trial worked, we would drop the placebo and whoever was HIV positive in Soweto in the future and was pregnant, I would make sure that there will be drugs [available]. We started then getting AZT from donations and making sure of rolling out an AZT program, so that was our promise to the women we worked with, and I'm glad to say, we've kept our promise. We gave AZT illegally to pregnant women from about 1998. We got people who were giving us donations and we got money to buy AZT. People would come and bring us bottles of AZT. Eventually, we got permission to provide AZT here.

The promise exacted from Gray, in fact, represented the ethical foundation for the clinical trial of which the women were part. The assumption was that, if effective, short-course AZT would become available in the public sector. All too soon, however, events would make clear that that was not to be the case. When the trial was brought to a conclusion in 1997, it was evident that the less costly regimen was effective in reducing the transmission of HIV from pregnant women to their babies. Nevertheless, South Africa's minister of health, Nkosazana Zuma, rejected the

possibility of making such treatment available. "I have to look at the whole picture. If you have limited resources, you may decide to put your resources into
preventing mothers getting infected in the first place. These are difficult issues we
have to face."[7] Those opposed to her position noted that, given the cost of the new
regimen as compared to the cost of treating babies with AIDS, not to speak of the
suffering and ultimate death of infected children, the new interventions clearly
passed the test of cost-benefit analysis.[8]

At a public meeting, Glenda Gray confronted the health minister, who had
avoided answering a direct question on whether the government would provide
AZT to pregnant women.

> I went and approached her, and I said, "You didn't answer the question.
> Are you going to give AZT to pregnant women?" And she said, "It's not
> cost effective." I said, "That is rubbish." And then we had a huge fight, and
> she said, "Don't tell me what to do. And it's not rubbish."

When Nkosazana Zuma was replaced as minister of health by Manto Tshabalala-
Msimang after Mbeki's presidential election in 1999, Gray's hopes rose. She had
known of the new minister's return from exile and thought of her as a "progressive."
But she was quickly disappointed. "Very soon, it was evident that it was going to be
as difficult to work with her as it had been with Zuma. They were digging in their
heels on mother-to-child transmission."

This was the context within which the grassroots Treatment Action Campaign
(TAC) was founded in December 1998. Its first action involved a demonstration in
Cape Town on December 10, Human Rights Day. One of its early leaders was
Zackie Achmat, a charismatic, gay, former anti-apartheid activist, who would become the internationally known spokesperson for the movement.[9] Among those
who would join him in this effort was Mark Heywood, a 34-year-old Nigerian-
born, white human rights activist whose early years in the anti-apartheid struggle
had been framed by his left-wing commitments. As the director of the AIDS Law
Project—an organization founded by Edwin Cameron that sought to use legal
redress to protect people with AIDS from discrimination—Heywood believed a
focus on treatment access was a natural and essential extension of his work. "You
can get someone their job back," he said in 2003, "but if they are not going to get
treatment, their lifestyle doesn't look that rosy." Looking back on TAC's efforts in
1998–1999, he recalled:

> We decided that our first campaign would be to try to persuade the South
> African government to use AZT. We did that because we thought pre-
> venting mother-to-child transmission was understandable to people who
> didn't have any concept that you could do anything medically about
> HIV. We wanted to break that notion. We did it, secondly, because we
> wanted to make a breakthrough and wanted to prevent infant infections

and prevent the pain that parents would suffer. We collected 50,000 signatures from communities. This was the first time that the activist movement did not go solely to professionals. We went out to all people and trade unions and explained the issues and got the signatures and began the movement. On March 21, 1999, we held demonstrations at Baragwanath Hospital, and in Durban and Cape Town. It was the first time that there had been demonstrations around access to treatment.

As they pressed their case, Heywood and Zackie Achmat increasingly were viewed by the minister of health and the office of President Mbeki as traitors to the ANC, to which they both belonged. At a meeting to discuss the government's policy, the minister of health denounced Heywood, whose life had once been threatened by the apartheid regime, as a "sellout." Heywood, who had suffered the loss of two infants, sought to underscore the human costs of the government's intransigence.

I just thought, "Screw this woman. If you think you are going to do this to me. . . . Well, I will make people understand in this meeting what the human side of this thing is." And so I said, "We are talking about a lot of women. We are not talking about statistics. We are not talking about a program. We are talking about women who have to go through childbirth knowing the risk to their children and then live with HIV-infected children."

Resistance to the government's stance took other forms as well. In at least one instance, a public hospital decided to provide AZT to pregnant women. Ashraf Coovadia, a pediatrician at Coronation Hospital in Johannesburg, recounted his hospital's efforts and open defiance, which included a published statement in the *South African Medical Journal*.[10]

The Coronation Hospital board took the decision that any mother that gets delivered here who is positive would get AZT. And they were getting AZT. This flew in the face of government, and so they took the brave and bold decision, until they got rapped on the knuckles and were told, "No, you can't do that. AZT is too toxic; it's not proven."

When a Ugandan trial[11] of the antiretroviral drug nevirapine demonstrated in 1999 that a single dose to the mother during delivery, followed by a dose to her child, could reduce maternal-fetal transmission—an intervention that was clearly affordable—the government balked again.[12] The Baragwanath neonatologist Haroon Saloojee recalled his initial sense of excitement, followed by a dawning appreciation of the depths of the government's resistance.

My first response was, Is this really possible? It sounds too good to be true. We waited for the reports and went through them, and said, "This sounds plausible. It sounds like you can really do it." There was an enormous excitement, because we suddenly realized that, finally, this can reduce mother-to-child transmission by half. Clearly now, the Health Department has no argument. They'll see the merit of this. I'm sure that within three months we are going to have nevirapine in all our hospitals. Nothing happened. Then the government argued that this was a Ugandan study and not a South African trial, and we needed a study done under South African conditions. I remember really thinking that we were wasting our time, but maybe that's what we needed to do. It was the first time that I got this impression of the government's opposition to drugs, to antiretrovirals.

At the conclusion of the South African nevirapine study in 2000, the government decided that it would only go forward with two pilot sites in each of the nation's nine provinces, thereby reaching an estimated 10 percent of women who delivered each year. In another act of defiance, Coronation Hospital decided to provide nevirapine. According to Ashraf Coovadia:

We had stocks of the drug, and it was Obstetric Department policy to continue to give mothers the nevirapine. We from the pediatric side felt the duty to follow up these children and that was the origin of our mother-to-child clinic. In effect, many of the people in the provincial Health Department just turned a blind eye, because they knew it was the right thing, so they just let us do it.

The government's decision to restrict access to nevirapine to 18 sites, and its rejection in July 2000 of the offer by Boehringer Ingelheim, the drug's manufacturer, to make it available free of charge for five years, further galvanized physicians and the Treatment Action Campaign.[13] After having been more cautious than some believed necessary, TAC made the decision to take the government to court, charging it with violating the constitutional right to health care when costs were not beyond the capacity of the state. Haroon Saloojee, who with Ashraf Coovadia had founded the organization Save Our Babies, agreed to serve as TAC's first complainant in court papers. "I saw my name as being the first applicant listed after the Treatment Action Campaign and had to make an immediate decision. As a government employee, was I willing to expose myself to this? It didn't take me too long to decide that this was the right thing to do."

Paralleling the development of its legal case, TAC continued to mobilize its constituency through demonstrations that eventuated in rallies and marches on November 25–26, 2001, just prior to the court hearing in Pretoria. On December 14, the High Court handed down its decision, a sharp rebuke of the government's policy. "A countrywide mother-to-child transmission program is an ineluctable obligation of the state."[14] The reliance on pilot studies was rejected because it entailed "no unqualified commitment to reach the rest of the population in any given time or at any given rate."[15] The government denounced the court decision as a usurpation of its authority to make policy for the nation. Indeed the ANC's Youth League gave voice to the sense of outrage.

> Judges are not elected to govern the country. They are not qualified to make political decisions about government, not to mention prescribing policies to the people's government. We wonder, Why does the court reduce itself to become an agent to drum up profits for multinational pharmaceutical companies whose only interest is to make money out of sick people?[16]

With the High Court decision providing a legal and moral context, provincial health authorities began to break ranks with the national government. The Western Cape Province, within which Cape Town is located, had already begun to extend its mother-to-child transmission efforts and hoped that by mid-2002 90 percent of pregnant women in the province would have access to such services.[17] In KwaZulu-Natal, the government decided in January 2002 to make nevirapine available to all pregnant women within the next two months.[18] The province's premier used the occasion to denounce the national government's position.

> The program of administering nevirapine would be warranted even if there were a small number of innocent lives to be saved, such is the elementary moral fact that the sovereign value of life is a fundamental right under the constitution and therefore imposes the principal obligation to act upon any responsible government.[19]

This apparently abrupt decision took clinicians in the province by surprise. Neil McKerrow, who had long recognized the need to provide HIV preventive services to pregnant women, underscored the importance of caution, even as he welcomed the reversal of official policy.

> We had to plan a response to the KwaZulu-Natal cabinet. What was quite interesting was that it was the clinicians who were saying, "We are not ready." We thought, we have got to get the infrastructure right. We've got to make sure that there is effective counseling, that there is effective infant feeding practices. Otherwise, if we went ahead, it would be a nonsustainable intervention. That's why, although the instruction came from the politicians, the actual implementation was delayed quite a while.

McKerrow then described a phase-in that extended over six months.

> It was phased in as the hospitals demonstrated that they were able to do it, and to do that meant they had the capacity for effective voluntary counseling. So they had to have privacy, a place where the patients wouldn't

be identified. They had to have the staff who had the skills and the time. So each hospital was given, if they didn't have space, a prefab building. They were given additional lay counselors. The nursing staff were taught to do the rapid HIV test. Someone was taught to discuss infant feeding practices. And we established basic midwifery practices and follow-up procedures for the babies. And when those were in place in each hospital, the antiretrovirals were introduced.

Just how important such infrastructural factors could be was underscored by Bernhard Gaede, whose role as the medical manager of Emmaus Hospital in KwaZulu-Natal made him acutely sensitive to practical limitations. Despite the availability of nevirapine, before the provincial government had moved forward with its own program, women had not been willing to get tested, the first step to discovering whether or not they were infected. In part, the issue was the quality of counseling. But more important were the "humongous" implications for women of knowing they were infected. At a hospital where approximately one-third of pregnant women were infected and which had over 100 deliveries a month, only 2–3 percent had taken nevirapine in 2003.

In July 2002, South Africa's Constitutional Court upheld the High Court decision handed down seven months earlier, giving an additional foundation to a process that was already well under way. "The policy of confining Nevirapine to research and training sites," said the court:

> fails to address the needs of mothers and their newborns and children. It fails to distinguish between the evaluation of programs for reducing mother-to-child transmission and the need to provide access to health care services required by those who do not have access to the sites.[20]

Despite the court's decision, there were provinces that, because of political loyalties to the president and his minister of health, adamantly refused to provide nevirapine.[21] Nevertheless, the tide had begun to shift. While the *Mail and Guardian* reported in mid-2003 that the mother-to-child transmission program was a "shambles" in six of South Africa's nine provinces—the exceptions being Gauteng, KwaZulu-Natal, and Western Cape[22]—it was possible in 2004 for TAC's Mark Heywood to say, "There is quite a wide availability of nevirapine now. It's imperfect in many respects. But imperfection is correctable." Jerry Coovadia, who had been a long-time, and often bitter, critic of the government's AIDS policies, was also uncharacteristically optimistic. "It's going to be a totally manageable issue. I think mother-to-child is solved."

But however important and however long in coming, he knew that this achievement was of limited significance. Mother-to-child transmission was, said Coovadia, "of course not the main driver of the epidemic." His epidemiological observation had a moral dimension as well, one that would fuel the next phase of the struggle for extending access to treatment, which would focus on mothers. As an obstetrician at King Edward VIII, Hannah Sebitloane, who had been taught by Coovadia, was troubled by the implications of the nevirapine victory.

> We always say that our first patient is the pregnant woman and not the baby. But we are just using the nevirapine to get to the baby. It's doing nothing for the mother. Sometimes I ask myself, what are we doing, having a beautiful baby who has no mother?

For TAC, which had always understood the initial focus on saving babies from HIV as but the prelude to a broader struggle, the time was ripe for an expanded campaign. "We would like to make mother-to-child transmission a battle of the past so we can fight to save HIV positive parents and continue the campaign for access to affordable and lifesaving medicines."[23]

Already those whose efforts were underwritten by charitable and international humanitarian organizations had taken steps to do just that. Linda-Gail Bekker and Robin Wood had successfully approached the British charity CRUSADE for funds to launch a mother-to-child transmission service in Guguletu, but they had to shift the focus of their appeal once the Western Cape provincial government decided to provide nevirapine.

> We went back to the funders and said, "Could we put on the table treatment for mothers, and if we are going to treat mothers, we would like to treat their partners, so can we put in a bid for treatment for families?" They liked it. We called it our family clinic. We decided that we would use women as the point of entry wherever possible, but if we found an index patient, we would look for the family.

The Western Cape Health Department agreed to pay for the infrastructure because it could not, given national policy, provide funds for antiretrovirals. CRUSADE agreed to underwrite the cost of treating 150 people for a year. Within six weeks, the clinic roster was filled. "We were overwhelmed," said Bekker. "One hundred and fifty cases was a drop in the ocean." She understood the need to increase the resources she could call on and began "fundraising like mad. Anybody who listened, I talked to them about drugs."

Also in the Western Cape, in the township of Khayelitsha, a major international humanitarian relief organization, Médecins sans Frontières (Doctors without Borders), winner of the Nobel Peace Prize in 1999, was pioneering an antiretroviral effort. MSF sought to demonstrate that both the medical and administrative obstacles so often invoked as reasons for not providing ART would yield if there was a commitment to treat the most needy.

Médecins sans Frontières

It was the prospect of launching a program to prevent mother-to-child transmission of HIV that initially brought Médecins sans Frontières and Eric Goemaere, then a 45-year-old doctor, to South Africa in 1999. MSF had been founded in 1971 by physicians who had worked in Biafra under the auspices of the Red Cross during the Nigerian civil war of the late 1960s. Disillusioned with the Red Cross's policy of not publicly revealing abuses and maintaining neutrality during that conflict, the doctors created an organization that offered emergency and long-term health care to populations affected by epidemics or earthquakes, wars or endemic poverty. But MSF also chose to bear witness to human rights abuses suffered by the people it treated, with the intent of publicizing its findings and bringing them to the attention of international bodies and national governments. For speaking out, it earned both praise and enmity (as was the case in Chechnya and Sudan), and had been expelled from a number of countries. Since 1999, MSF had extended its commitment to reducing obstacles to effective clinical care, notably by campaigning on behalf of people in poorer countries to overcome the financial and logistical barriers to essential medicines for common infectious diseases. These included effective drugs for tuberculosis, malaria, and HIV/AIDS.[24]

Eric Goemaere, MSF's former medical director, admitted that it had come late to AIDS, but argued that HIV prevention focused on population-wide education and condom distribution could be more effectively accomplished by governments. With the discovery that antiretrovirals reduced mother-to-child transmission, MSF realized that it could at last provide an important clinical service to poor populations. MSF and Goemaere, who had studied Marxist economics before turning to medicine, were also drawn to the events unfolding in South Africa, where, they believed, the government was taking on the large Western pharmaceutical firms, the United States, and several European countries in order to reduce the costs of antiretroviral medications. (The dispute centered on South Africa's Medicines and Related Substances Control Amendment Act of 1997, which authorized compulsory "fast track" drug licensing and the parallel importation of cheaper medicines when necessary to protect the public's health.)[25] Goemaere recalled:

> I thought South Africa would be a symbolic country, because it was 1999
> and the International AIDS Conference, to be held in Durban, was coming a
> year later. We would be able to show something could be done to the world
> conference. I thought it would be extremely simple. South Africa, being
> the country with the highest amount of infected people, would be interested
> naturally in treatment, and it would be in the forefront—as they already
> were among the nonaligned nations—fighting for access to antiretrovirals.

Goemaere planned to situate his effort in Alexandra, a historically impoverished township near Johannesburg, which had been the site of a now-famous community health program inspired by Sidney and Emily Kark's work, which had offered primary health care while involving community members in its operations.[26] After 1948, the newly elected apartheid government put an end to the Karks' program. Now it was a government composed of veterans of the anti-apartheid struggle that sought to quash Goemaere's effort. "Unfortunately, Alexandra is very close to the Department of Health in Pretoria," said Goemaere. "And when I went to Pretoria to announce this idea, they told me clearly that antiretroviral therapy was not part of the public sector package and that I was not allowed to use anti-retrovirals." His mission blocked, Goemaere decided to go elsewhere. Before leaving South Africa, he visited with TAC's Zackie Achmat, with whom he had been in correspondence. Achmat, who lived in the Western Cape, which was more open to treating people with HIV, alerted him to possibilities.

> Zackie told me, "Hang on, I think they started something in Khayelitsha."
> I discovered that, in fact, the provincial minister for health, an ANC guy, had taken the decision in defiance of the national government to start a MTCT [mother-to-child transmission] program there. They had started it confidentially. It took me a month to convince them of the interest of MSF to be here, because they thought I was certainly going to make a lot of noise about it. Then the whole thing would collapse, because they would know about it at the national level.

As Goemaere surveyed the existing MTCT program in Khayelitsha, a township of a half million people, he found that it was shrouded in secrecy and staffed by ill-trained nurses. His response was to address the conditions that were hobbling the effort.

> I spent months going around interviewing the nurses, trying to see what could be done, and even the ones in the MTCT program were extremely negative. Those nurses were confusing HIV infection with terminal AIDS, because that's the only thing they could see. They weren't testing at that time. The nurses felt, "This disease is not a threat for me. But I am a midwife here, and this bloody program is bringing to me those few individuals that are infected. I am going to get infected with that." We had to do training, a lot of training, to explain HIV and AIDS to everybody.

Through these efforts, said Goemaere, dramatic changes began to occur.

> They started slowly to understand: I am only seeing the tip of the iceberg. There are between 40 and 50,000 infected people here in Khayelitsha; it's everywhere, HIV is everywhere. Probably it's in my family as well, even if I am a nurse or a midwife. I am not protected against it. It's better to have a proactive attitude.

By 2000, the annual HIV survey of Khayelitsha's antenatal clinics estimated that almost 20 percent of pregnant women were infected. Two years later, the MTCT program, which tested 95 percent of pregnant women, found that 25 percent were seropositive.[27] Voluntary counseling and testing in the township's tuberculosis, family planning, and sexually transmitted disease services revealed that 31 percent of those tested were positive. In addition to the high prevalence rates, among the highest in the Western Cape, what was striking to Goemaere was that people in Khayelitsha were stepping forward to be tested. MSF's approach to providing comprehensive HIV care was, he believed, crucial to the change he was witnessing.

> Why is MSF convinced that it has to initiate antiretroviral treatment? Of course, for a humanitarian reason, because you cannot let people die in such a scandalous way. But also because we strongly believe that it will change totally the relation the people have with that disease.

What had begun with prevention of mother-to-child transmission was, in May 2001, extended by MSF to assure that the mothers of babies born HIV-free should themselves survive. "The child survives, but we are producing orphans here. So let's make the mothers survive."

But MSF's vision of what needed to be done went beyond the treatment of mothers. It sought to demonstrate that ART could be effectively used in a primary care setting to treat an impoverished population. The effort did not begin without a struggle between Goemaere and the provincial Health Department. In South Africa, the provinces are permitted to define their own health priorities as long as they don't conflict with those of the national government. Ultimately, MSF was permitted to extend its program after both sides had agreed upon a subterfuge to forestall interference from Pretoria.

> The provincial authorities thought, This is going to put us in trouble with the national government, so it was a long discussion. I said, "It's part of the deal. If you tell me no antiretrovirals, I am gone." Finally, we made an agreement, which was that the use of antiretrovirals was private research by MSF, operational research. And, as operational research, you are entitled to do almost whatever you want, as long as you have ethics committee approval. So it was playing a little bit with the words.

As it began its efforts, MSF understood it needed to procure low-priced drugs. It had first turned to the Western pharmaceutical giants—GlaxoSmithKline, Boehringer Ingelheim, and Hoffmann–La Roche—to determine whether they would sell their medications at the prices set by the manufacturers of generic drugs. They uniformly refused. Glaxo offered to make a small-scale donation, which Goemaere felt he had to reject. "We thought," Goemaere said, "with a small-scale donation, we don't demonstrate anything, because this will be a demonstration for myself. What about the country?" Although strategically correct, Goemaere felt ethically troubled by his actions, which postponed the day he could prescribe antiretroviral drugs and all but assured that patients would die who might have lived.

> In 2000, we treated a lot of opportunistic infections, and those people were inevitably dying. I was thinking, Do I take my patients hostage? Why don't I buy those drugs, even at full price? I am a representative of an international organization that is extremely rich. Do I not breach my Hippocratic oath—which says you are obliged to do the maximum that you can do for your patient—by not providing them with antiretrovirals? And I haven't solved that question.

The poignancy and delicacy of that moral choice was never clearer than when the chief executive officer of Boehringer Ingelheim, Africa, came to visit Khayelitsha.

> The guy accepted to come to Khayelitsha. He saw this little child, an orphan, who usually came with his grandmother, but that day he was alone, nine years old, dying from AIDS. And that's exactly what I wanted, to make him be confronted with the reality, what we were facing here. And he said, "Can I pay for treatment for this child personally?"

Goemaere's impulse was to say, "No, that's not the point here; the point is not only this child. There are thousands of them. If we come to an agreement for reducing the price of the drugs, of course you can pay for the treatment of this child." Instead, he responded, "Yes, we can discuss it." He continued, "The point here is, I didn't want to make this child hostage of that deal. I would never do that. Unfortunately, the child died shortly afterwards, and we didn't come to an agreement about reducing the price."

In September 2001, Goemaere got permission from the national government's Medicines Control Council to use generic antiretrovirals imported from Brazil. Although he had feared that the pharmaceutical companies would act to block MSF's use of such drugs, he believed that international opinion and shareholder pressures helped to stay the industry's hand.

> The pharmaceutical companies had all the legal right to attack us in court, and worse, to call for the seizure of the drugs. We were very nervous. I believe that the pharmaceutical companies understood—it was a large debate in front of the world, including their shareholders—that this is not acceptable. We all need to make this work. We don't speak about Viagra here.

MSF began its ART program slowly, then accelerated its efforts. One hundred patients were enrolled in the program by the end of 2001, 300 by the end of the following year. By January 2004, 776 patents were in treatment, 84 of them children. Although the Mbeki government did not block the MSF-provincial anti-retroviral program, the media were used to vilify Goemaere's motives and his use of such drugs. Government representatives likened Eric Goemaere and the MSF to a notorious, racist chemist and biological warfare scientist in the employ of the apartheid regime.

> We have been accused in the media. During 1999 and 2000, there was a regular statement about the toxicity of AZT used in the MTCT program. We got patients coming to us to say, "Doctor, have you heard what they said on the radio from the national Department of Health? Is it really toxic?" The worst attack that we got was when we started with triple therapy in May 2001, where Smuts Ngonyama, a spokesperson of the ANC, wrote in the newspaper here that we were fighting with biological warfare. He was implying that we were a modern version of Wouter Basson, who was the Dr. Mengele here during apartheid, who was doing experiments to develop racist dogs and all sorts of experiments to sterilize Black people. We didn't react directly. We sent a delegation of 20 patients, and they went to see him, and they told him, "We are not dead, we are alive, you can see, so you are going to retract your words. You are the criminal." He never apologized publicly.

Goemaere's status as a foreigner who favored ART served to fuel the attacks by those who charged him with being party to an international plot headed by the pharmaceutical companies. He found ongoing political support in the Treatment Action Campaign and in the clinics' patients, who were sometimes themselves the ground troops of TAC.

> So we are in the middle of a political war. TAC is doing the job, an enormous job. Within TAC, most of them are HIV positive. Several of them are clients, and today they are alive because they have been treated. And they do the political work here. Some people say that this is worse than apartheid. Health, it's an obsession here, because people are dying all over. And they don't understand why this government doesn't want to do for them what could easily be done.

Through TAC, Goemaere also found an ally in Nelson Mandela, who publicly attached himself to the cause of AIDS treatment in Khayelitsha. In 2002, Zackie Achmat brought them together. "That was the dream of my life, to meet this guy, and he called me Eric." Goemaere recalled that Mandela confided, "In my own country, to get an appointment with my successor, President Mbeki, it's so difficult. And when I finally get him on the phone, he comes with all those technical arguments, and I am not a doctor." Goemaere then said to him:

"Mr. President, do me a favor, come to Khayelitsha. You don't need to be a doctor, because I don't think the president of the country has to play as if he was a doctor. Keep to principles, and the principle is, when you can afford it, give treatment and give hope to this young democracy." And that's what Mandela understood very well.

In a visit both public and strategic, the former president, combining political astuteness and his immense personal charisma, demonstrated what separated him from his successor.

He came in December 2002, this powerful person inside the ANC coming to visit our particular program. We thought that the most strong symbol would be if he could wave this "HIV Positive" T-shirt, which is the symbol of all the political fights here for access to treatment. It was given to him by our very first patient who got antiretrovirals in May 2001. And there was Madiba magic, as they say; he is called "Madiba" in this country. Within a second, the guy, in front of everybody, took his shirt off and put the T-shirt on. He was wearing it in front of all the cameras, this "HIV Positive" T-shirt.

Thus, recalled Goemaere, Mandela linked his image as the leader of the struggle against apartheid, his smile and wave, with those who had a despised and stigmatized disease. He had associated his presence in the township with the life-saving provision of antiretrovirals to its Black inhabitants.

The introduction of ART for the treatment of AIDS was transformative for both patients and clinical staff in Khayelitsha. Sister Veliswa Labatala, a 30-year-old nurse, raised in the township where she worked, first came to the MSF HIV clinic with suspicions that Black patients were serving as antiretroviral guinea pigs. A chance encounter with a woman she believed had died, crystallized for her the benefits of ART.

I was young and wanted to know more about HIV, and fortunately for me, around about 2002, there was a post with MSF to work in one of their HIV/AIDS clinics. To be quite honest, I was much more interested in knowing, what are these people here to do? They are going to work with our people, our Black community—why us? During that time, there was so much negativity from the government. If they are using Black people as guinea pigs, as a staunch member of ANC, I had to know. I had to get the information, and, if it's true, then expose them. If not, I wanted to be one of the people that would mobilize our Black community.

When I came on board, there were patients that I had been seeing in my previous chronic diseases clinics that I thought were dead because of their HIV condition. One of them must have come into MSF—and she was bad, she was just bedridden. She would be carried from a stretcher to a wheelchair, from a wheelchair to the bed. And this lady that I'm telling you about had been admitted to a TB hospital. She disappeared.

I was busy in the MSF clinic one day because it was full. There was this lady who kept calling my name and saying, "Look at me." I thought, "She's really annoying me." She was beautiful, plump, makeup on, and I said to her, "I do see you. What do you want?" She said, "Don't you know me?" And I thought, "Please, not now," because I grew up in Khayelitsha and I know most people who would come in. So I said, "But I'm working here. Can I first finish? Then I'll come to you." She said, "No, I don't want to wait. Remember me? I used to be in the wheelchair." The clinic doctor told me she was on antiretrovirals. I said, "I could not recognize her!" And we hugged. Right then, we sang. Others sang. Then, "Shhhh! We're still in hospital." And now the other people were looking at us, and she said, "Yes, I have HIV!" She went around and she told people, and she said, "I was almost dying. Actually, I was a walking corpse. I am on antiretrovirals, and look!" And she was weighing 35 kilograms then, and now she's weighing about 80 something. I thought, This is working. That then convinced me about ART. I stopped being skeptical. I just wanted to go for it.

For Eric Goemaere, the work in Khayelitsha involved more than the management of clinics. He had become a practicing doctor and formed close professional relationships with patients. Previously, like most MSF physicians, Goemaere had served for less than a year, sometimes only for months, in horrific settings like Chechnya, the Congo, and Rwanda. He had usually provided services or managed large groups following disasters. "The difference is," Goemaere said, "you are treating them collectively. You don't establish a relationship with them, you don't know them." Now, he was treating individuals. "Patients that come regularly, and you start to know them very well and you start to know the families." The failure of ART, Goemaere recalled, when it happened, cut all the more painfully.

The patients on antiretrovirals, they reinvent a sort of special life. People have decided they will die. Here, you see people dying from AIDS, so there's no doubt that it's a deadly disease. And suddenly, they discover that there's a life after death, because whoop, they are going up again. So they reopen this old world of possibilities, like an adolescent. And when they collapse again, that's terrible.

Goemaere, who had seen so many anonymous deaths as an MSF worker, was emotionally shaken as he recounted the story of a patient who died despite careful and attentive care.

I remember a 24-year-old guy, his name is James, who was attacked by a very vicious form of Norwegian scabies. It was horrible. He had skin like a

lizard from top to the bottom, very thick. It's a permanent deforma-
tion, and it's painful because it's cracked everywhere, gets so infected, and
it's extremely itchy. The family couldn't stand it any more and had decided to put him at the Sisters of Mercy hospice. It's where you are sent to
die. At least, with the incredible job they do, they die with a little bit of
dignity. It is, in other words, the dumping grounds where the families who
do not want to hear about the disease put the relative. But the mother
was still bringing him to the consultation; that's how he appeared the first
time.

This poor guy couldn't stay in front of me. He was oozing, and he
could hardly engage in a conversation. The mother was answering for him.
And you don't rush with antiretrovirals. You first have to stabilize him, so
step by step I managed to. He had not only diarrhea, he had TB of the
esophagus, and a terrible peripheral neuropathy. His main problem was
this itchy skin. He was literally like a lizard so he didn't look very human
any more. All the time itchy, crying, this guy was crying, and a guy at
24 crying, it's hard, it's something that is not easy to stand. He just wanted
to give up. And that was part of the reason why the family was giving up.
And I could, with time, clean his skin to a point that he felt almost comfortable. More important, he started to look like a human being. And
the mother decided to take him back, and we readmitted him amongst, not
only the human society, but even amongst the family. In itself, that was
an achievement. It took me weeks and weeks to do that.

We had long discussions whether or not to put him on ART. His CD4
count, as far as I remember, was less than 5. The problem you have with
treating late like that is that you have terrible reconstitution syndrome,
and unfortunately it was too late for him. He died two weeks after starting
the treatment. It was beyond change for him. I didn't see him when he
died. You swear and you are very cross, because you tried to see what you
did wrong. As a doctor, did I treat too late? What is the mistake I did?

News of the Khayelitsha HIV services and the existence there of antiretrovirals
filtered out into other townships and Black rural areas. With no treatment programs available to them, people with AIDS made their way to the MSF clinics with
the hope of finding assistance. The tragedy of their individual plights gripped
Goemaere, who remembered one particularly poignant case.

What was new for me is the way the patients look at you because they know
it's a deadly disease. Suddenly, they found something that might save
them. Some of them, they are coming from very far away. In fact, we would
only treat people from Khayelitsha.

I remember a young girl, 18 years old. She almost died on the consultation bed here. She was totally exhausted. She had traveled 1,200 kilometers

by taxi, because she had heard that there was a clinic somewhere around
Cape Town where there was a possibility to be treated. She had TB; she
had everything. And she looked at me, and she asked me, "Doctor, do I
have it?" She didn't speak that well, but it meant, "Do I have AIDS?"
She probably understood that, in a way, it was too late. "Do I still have
HIV? Do I have a chance?" Full-blown AIDS with esophageal thrush,
TB certainly, most of the symptoms; it was full-blown AIDS, and she was
still asking me, "Do I have AIDS?" You know the words mean, "Did I
arrive too late to you?" And the way she was questioning me, looking at me.
I got to cry a couple of times, which doesn't happen to me any more.

In the presence of such tragedies and in the absence of government programs,
MSF decided to expand its services to a poorer, less well medically served rural area
in the Eastern Cape. It was impelled to do so by the continued refusal of the government to provide antiretroviral therapy and what it saw as the official canard
that services of the level provided by MSF could not be replicated outside sophisticated urban centers like Cape Town. Hermann Reuter, a 37-year-old Namibian-
born doctor whose early ties to TAC led him to work for several years with Eric
Goemaere in Khayelitsha, said:

Our program in Khayelitsha was a success story, both in South African
medical circles and international media circles. But our government
was still looking for ways to dodge responsibility, and one of the arguments
that often came up was that Cape Town is urban, Cape Town has got a
good infrastructure. ART won't work in the rest of the country. On the
other hand, a lot of the patients we treated in Cape Town came from the
Eastern Cape and told us that in the Eastern Cape things are much worse,
and if MSF really wants to help, they should commit themselves to the
Eastern Cape. We chose the Eastern Cape because our patients pushed us.
[The] Eastern Cape is also politically the home ground of a lot of the ANC
heavyweights.

Financial support for this effort came through the Nelson Mandela Foundation, which had already funded schools there. Anxious to leave for a rural setting,
Reuter accepted Goemaere's offer to head the new venture. With MSF colleagues,
he settled on Lusikisiki, an area of 150,000 inhabitants, deep in the Transkei, as the
site for HIV medical care.

I wanted to leave Cape Town desperately. I was sick and tired of city life.
We looked at six districts that had hospitals that were ready to start
ART. Lusikisiki was one of the districts. And I knew Lusikisiki because
during my student days I went hiking there, and I liked the area. So,
emotionally, I thought it should be Lusikisiki. And we also got a warm

reception there, and so everybody agreed. HIV has got a very high prevalence there, because the mines recruit a lot of people from the area; and
because of the migrant labor, there's a higher infection rate there than in
other rural areas of the Eastern Cape. Politically, the people there are
ANC, but they are not just Mbeki followers; they are a bit independent
from the rest, and I thought, politically, that might be advantageous. So
everything fitted together; it just had to be Lusikisiki.

Among Reuter's first steps was to hire HIV counselors and reach out to hire
nurses at primary care sites who would provide the backbone of his initiative. He
was stunned by the flood of people who came forward for testing.

In the first week, I visited all the clinics, just to introduce myself to nurses,
because I knew in my mind it had to be a clinic-based program, not a
hospital-based model. It had to be primary health care at the clinics. And so
I went to see the 12 clinics of Lusikisiki, and I spoke to the nurses: "I will
show you how to test people, and you can talk with them." So we did a
workshop to teach nurses to do rapid tests, because before testing was only
done at hospitals for the inpatients that were sick. There was a *big* interest
in testing in the community. The first day, I sat with the nurses doing
the HIV testing, just to supervise them. It was the day when pensions were
paid out, so all these pensioners came for the HIV test. I didn't think many
of these people had HIV, but for the community to accept HIV, it's
probably important that I test the people that come. So we started testing
them. Eventually, we found a man, more than 70 years, HIV positive. The
next time I came to that clinic, two weeks later, the whole place was full of
school students. "We are coming for an HIV test. The teachers told us to
take off from school if we come for an HIV test." So you start. Testing,
testing, testing. Two of those students tested positive.
    And the motives for testing were not clear, but there was interest in
testing. A lot of widows: "My husband died in the mines, so I think he
might have been HIV positive." The other thing is that politicians in the
Eastern Cape had said that people with HIV can get a disability grant. We
tested more than 600 people the first month. It was amazing.

By 2005, the 12 clinics were testing 1,200 people a month. The infection rate was 42
percent.
    But despite such enthusiasm, the MSF effort in Lusikisiki was radically limited
by provincial politics, which were far more restrictive than those of the Western
Cape. On his arrival in Lusikisiki, Reuter was able to establish a prevention program
for pregnant women that used nevirapine. But the provincial Health Department
forbade him from using antiretroviral drugs as ongoing treatment for AIDS. He
was thus limited to preparing for the day when he might do so.

Corporate Interest, Corporate Responsibility: Anglo American's Embrace of Antiretroviral Therapy

That MSF would challenge the refusal of South Africa's government to provide life-saving treatment to people with HIV disease was no surprise. Far different was the decision of Anglo American, one of South Africa's most prestigious corporations, a pillar of its economy with links to international capital, and the employer of over 125,000 people in southern Africa.[28] The determination to provide antiretrovirals free of charge to its miners, most of whom were migrant laborers, was all the more striking, given the corporation's labor history and its early response to AIDS.[29] Involved is a story of how its vice president for medical affairs, Brian Brink, would move over time, to advocate not only for Anglo American's responsibility to its workers, but for government efforts to extend treatment to all who needed it. In marshaling appeals to corporate self-interest and benevolence, he was joined by another ardent advocate for reform, Gavin Churchyard, a physician and epidemiologist born in 1958 in what is today Zambia, who had tracked with growing alarm the rising toll of HIV among miners.

After attending the 1996 International AIDS Conference in Vancouver, Canada, where data about the efficacy of antiretrovirals had seized the imagination of delegates, radically transforming the pessimism that had for years surrounded the treatment of AIDS, Churchyard was convinced that ART would have to be incorporated into the health care system operated by the mines. Looking back in 2003, he said:

> I realized that because of the complexities then of the treatment regimens and particularly because of the costs, it wasn't affordable to the industry at that point in time. I started doing a lot of presentations, talking at congresses and to groups around TB control and just describing what was happening within our environment. From 1996, I had a slide which was called "ART: Not Yet, but Watch This Space." And for me, it was a case, not *if* ART became available; it was merely the case of *when* ART became available. At that time, it was absolutely rejected. No one was prepared to consider it. My approach was that penicillin, when it was first introduced, was also extremely expensive and only the most affluent people had access to penicillin. Today, the poorest country in the world has penicillin. So I was very aware that we needed to constantly have in mind that antiretroviral therapy would become available; everything I did from then on was working towards that goal.
>
> For me, it was the one thing that gave hope. I certainly wasn't prepared to accept that this would not be available in resource-limited settings. Things change because we make them change. And how do you change them? You engage, you talk, you push, you demand.

For the miner whose AIDS had progressed, in the absence of ART, to the point where he could no longer work, the end of employment generally meant the termination of all company-sponsored medical care and "repatriation." In that regard, AIDS was no different from end-stage renal disease. Like miners with AIDS, as one doctor noted, "That was another death sentence. They would die in time, and there was always the agony of discussing it with the patients and making them well aware of what was going on and how best to deal with it."

Both Churchyard and Brian Brink were determined to effect a change, so that, as in the case of tuberculosis, HIV positive miners could be treated, maintained, and successfully sent back to work. But the road to reform, both men found, would be painfully slow. Brink, as a senior executive, understood that his appeal would have to pass the cost-benefit threshold that defined the world view of corporate leaders.

> It's been interesting dealing with businessmen who are in the natural resources business. They know how to run mines, and they know how to take risks. They will risk huge sums of money on business ventures. Because they understand the business, they know the risks they're exposed to. They know how to manage and deal with them. When it comes to health care issues like AIDS, at the outset, they simply didn't understand it. They're unsure and they're uncertain. You spend time, as I have done, with them and explain, "This is a risk that we can quantify, that we can manage and fully understand." Then, you find the attitudes changing.

Churchyard, more the epidemiologist, turned to research to demonstrate the usefulness and viability of ART in the mines.

> Research was one way to change people's beliefs about what can be done, giving them the data and particularly the cost effectiveness. Within business, bottom lines, that's what talks. I became increasingly more passionate and obsessed with trying to make a difference. People often spoke of AIDS fatigue, of just being so overwhelmed by this constant burden of morbidity and mortality that you become totally disconnected from reality. I don't think that happened for me; it was a constant driving force to find ways of making a difference.
>
> So, when we introduced a wellness clinic, we started to provide preventive therapy, ongoing education, counseling. We conceived that this was the vehicle into which we were going to introduce ART when it became available. So we designed every system to accommodate ART. Back then, the companies weren't even prepared to consider it, but we designed our systems for it.

Like the International AIDS Conference in Vancouver, the 2000 International AIDS meeting in Durban, the first in a developing country, energized Churchyard.

Following the meeting "and the hype around antiretroviral therapy then, and the drive to make it more affordable," he attempted to convince the mining industry to consider ART seriously. Brink, in turn, had convinced the executive committee of Anglo American, toward the end of 2000, to approve a strategy document that included the goal of "finding ways and means to provide access to sustainable and affordable antiretroviral therapy for people progressing to AIDS." It was a move that was all the more striking given the increasingly vitriolic attacks by the government on antiretrovirals and those who advocated their use.

Because of the continued high cost of ART and other uncertainties, both men sought to employ operations research to move their campaign to the next stage. Unfortunately, rather than the straight path for which they had hoped, Brink confronted a series of sharply disappointing cul de sacs. Brink recalled:

Suddenly, the enormity of what it meant to provide ART began to dawn on managers—not only in terms of cost, which was prohibitive, but the infrastructure needed to do it. In 2001, what we were talking about was, well, we have to set it up on a smaller scale in a couple of places, learn how to do it properly, and then roll it out on a mass scale. We put together a whole pilot study, and during the course of putting it together, the name changed to a "feasibility study," which was almost a step backwards. The pilot implies, and I remember our chairman saying, "We don't do pilots with a view to failure, but with a view to success." And so we took a step back.

We had a study drawn up, much like a clinical trial, with an initial 2,000 participants. Then it was 1,250. There were long negotiations with drug companies about the extent to which we would be able to access affordable price breaks. The feasibility study eventually was finalized. I had that whole proposal, and I remember taking it to our executive almost as a formality, just to get the sign-off.

News of the corporate decision received not only local but international press attention. In mid-2001, South Africa's *Mail and Guardian* reported that the corporation planned to offer ART to its seropositive workforce, providing cost was not an obstacle—a matter that seemed to be resolved by Brink's observation, "The price of drugs has come down dramatically and at this stage, on balance, is in the realm of feasibility."[30] In the United States, the *Wall Street Journal* also reported the news, describing Anglo executives as hoping that their proposed use of ART would assure concerned investors that the company could limit the epidemic's effects.[31]

But what Brink had taken to be a settled matter soon began to unravel. At a meeting of corporate leaders, concerns about taking on too much of a burden dominated the discussions.

I couldn't believe it—they simply did not feel secure enough in the knowledge that what they were doing was right. And they said, "Look, we need to share this with some other people, take this to the broader mining industry, and get other mining groups to come and participate in this feasibility study. Do a feasibility study on the level of the trade association, the Chamber of Mines, not at Anglo American. It's too risky for us on our own. And bring the government in, and bring the trade unions in, and let everybody take their share of risk on this thing." And that was profoundly disappointing to me. I had been led to believe we were up and running. Suddenly, we took a whole step backward. And there were quite a few newspaper articles at the time. "Anglo does a U turn on its ART policy" and that sort of thing. I began to be very despondent with that.

The *Wall Street Journal*, which a year earlier had reported that corporate leaders saw in ART a way to face the impact of AIDS, now noted that concerns about financial risk dictated the very opposite course, given the cheapness of labor: "While the cost of the drugs in developing countries has plummeted, they remain expensive compared with the wages and benefits Anglo pays its low-skilled mineworkers."[32] Months earlier, as Anglo dragged its feet over ART to miners but made it available to salaried employees through their medical aid plans, the National Union of Mine Workers had charged it with racism and caring more for profits than for ordinary workers' lives.[33]

As Anglo American tried to "share its costs" with the rest of the mining industry, Brink was brought to the edge of despair. According to Brink:

Anglo took it to the Chamber of Mines and got all the other employers in. It was fascinating to watch that process, because we had envisaged a feasibility study with 1,200 participants, which would have been very costly. The discussion in the Chamber of Mines was, "Can't we trim it down a bit? We can do this with 600, not 1,200. Where you wanted to do it on six sites, we think we can do it on three sites." And it was all to make the cost of the feasibility study less. I remember thinking to myself, "What's the point? If you're serious about wanting to do ART for everybody, the cost of the feasibility study is trivial in comparison. This is just a way to postpone having to deal with the issue." So that whole process in the Chamber of Mines was hugely, hugely frustrating. You can imagine—just a time of huge despondency.

For Brink, the stunning collapse of his efforts led to a painful rethinking of his corporate identity. Unable to accept what he considered to be an ill-founded decision, at 50 years of age Brian Brink reluctantly decided to resign, a stand that he did not hide from his superiors.

When you work for an employer for 20 years, and then you're at a senior level, it's not easy to just get up and go. It's actually a good job. But

shortly after one of the meetings, when it had become clear that Anglo
backtracked on ART, I remember going to my supervisor and saying,
"We're now going in different directions, and we have to part company.
I cannot reconcile myself to what's happening here, and I'm telling
you now I'm looking around." Somewhat to my surprise, he told the chief
executive.

Anglo's chief executive responded to this challenge by making a commitment
to the support of community-based AIDS prevention efforts and vaccine initiatives.
But it was only after the International AIDS Meeting in Barcelona in June 2002 that
Anglo American's position on ART changed. During the conference, Coca Cola and
Anglo American were pilloried by activists for refusing to underwrite antiretroviral
drugs for their employees. Brink watched these activities with mixed emotions.

They had demonstrations every day. "Coke and Anglo, you can't hide! We
charge you with genocide!" They were singing this out with big Coke
bottles and placards. It was a peculiar feeling to watch it from the outside
and a tremendous tearing, of wanting to sympathize, and also wanting to
be loyal to the company at the same time.

On his return to South Africa, Brink had an extraordinary meeting with the
company's chief executive, who asked him to draft a paper immediately for the
company's executive committee on implementing ART throughout Anglo American. Shortly thereafter, in July 2002, a new policy was adopted, despite the corporation's history of repatriating unproductive workers and the claims of some
that it was cheaper to let workers die.

It was the most remarkable experience. It just went by so quickly. In any
big organization, you've got a lot of influential business people, heavy
hitters. You've got to get them all to think the same way. It becomes a hell
of a lot easier when the chief executive says, "This is what we're going to
do." I have to credit him for that; once he became convinced that this
was the right thing to do, it was unstoppable. The others there weren't sure.
The turnover of employees getting sick or dying from AIDS was actually
not that great; you're really talking about 3 percent per annum. Some of the
businessmen would simply say, "I can handle that. They can move on.
As they go, I'll replace them. I don't have to get involved paying exorbitant
amounts for ART. There's vast unemployment in this country, lots of
people wanting jobs. No big deal for us; we can just carry on."

For Brink, such views had become unconscionable. Despite his acknowledgment of
the importance of corporate cost-benefit considerations, the provision of ART was
now a moral imperative.

Everybody keeps asking us, "What's it going to cost?" as if it's a cost-benefit analysis. The decision was not based on economics—I mean, clearly, we looked at the economics—but far more important a thing was the social imperative, simply that people are dying. You cannot stand by and watch this epidemic taking root in this country and do nothing.

Despite his sense of social mission, Brink remained attentive to the logic of economics. He negotiated with the drug companies to obtain the lowest prices available in South Africa, those offered to public and nonprofit entities.

I know that these drugs are being made available in this country at a price of what was one-tenth of what you might have to pay in the First World. These are the prices available to governments and possibly the nongovernmental organizations. It was unheard-of that an employer might get access to this kind of pricing. But in the many discussions I had with them, I said, "Look, this is a disease that selectively targets economically active people, and if the economic engine of these developing countries starts to falter, then we will truly have a disaster—so your access programs need to extend." The drug companies are very perceptive. I had early indications that they would afford us that same opportunity of access to preferential pricing.

Whatever the ultimate reasons for Anglo's reversal—pressure from capital markets and shareholders in the United States and Britain, concern about the cost of international obloquy, the moral force of the arguments made by a trusted senior official—once it had decided to provide ART, it moved quickly, setting up nurse-centered clinics with a standardized treatment regimen in its eight divisions. Anglo American's Aurum Institute for Health Research distributed material, educated employees and management, trained medical staff, and developed uniform data recording, monitoring, and reporting systems. By November 2002, the first patients were placed on ART; a year later, the number stood at just over 1,000, a modest achievement that was still well below Brink's target of 3,000.

Brink understood that in an organization like Anglo American, management had to assume the responsibility for overcoming years of fear, stigma, and ignorance to convince the miners to come forward for counseling and testing. Thus, the shortfall represented a managerial failure. "In the context of the workplace, it's the mine managers. There are performance indicators which every operation has to report on a regular basis. And when we see unsatisfactory targets, we go back to the managers and say, 'That's not good enough.'"

There were positive examples that Brink could call upon as he dealt with his disappointment. Some local mine executives were very successful, harnessing their management teams, union representatives, and their own example to pull the rank and file into the health stations for HIV counseling and testing. He recalled:

In one of our mines, the new manager, from the day he arrived, made it his
personal crusade to increase the level of awareness and action around
AIDS. Part of his agenda was getting people to know their HIV status.
Within a period of six months, he had got 57 percent of his mine workforce
to voluntarily go and have an HIV test. And he was the first person in
the front row tested, along with the rest of his management. Every meeting
I've been to where we talk about AIDS, the head of the union is in there
right next to him. He's involved the union in the thing all the way.

But in the opinion of Kathryn Mngadi, chief of the HIV wellness clinic at
AngloGold's Orkney mine in 2004, the reluctance of miners to begin antiretroviral
treatment was often beyond the reach of individual managers, based on the limits
of their health care coverage.

There's a lot of concern among the miners that once they are not working
here—retrenchments, if they're fired, if they're too sick—they worry
that they won't be able to continue the treatment. You must remember our
preparation is about emphasizing that the treatment is lifelong. So a lot of
the guys feel, Well, unless you're going to treat me when I'm finished
working here, or there's a place that you can refer me to where I can access
the treatment for a reasonable cost, then what's the point?

Doctors employed by the mine hospitals and clinics to provide day-to-day
medical services also proved to be an impediment. These physicians, according to
Mngadi, retained their suspicion of specialist knowledge and an attitude toward
AIDS treatment that was a mixture of skepticism and paternalistic racism.

There's not a big eagerness, even though we have antiretrovirals, to refer
patients to the clinic. Or they'll refer them very late, when they've got them
in the ward and they've got multiple opportunistic infections, and they
think, What else can I do? And then they say, "Send them to Kathy!" A
gentleman on whom they made a diagnosis of AIDS dementia complex lay
there and deteriorated until he was in a vegetative state before I got to know
that he was there. I said, "Guys, I'm up the passage." I'm not sure if it's
because they don't have any experience of patients on antiretrovirals.
There's almost a suspicion—sort of, "Does it work? Really?" And there's a
lot of cynicism around miners taking antiretrovirals. "Oh, they'll default. There'll be resistance. They're infecting their wives." So those gen-
eralizations are really applied very broadly and very often by a lot of the
doctors.

Like Brink, the Treatment Action Campaign's Mark Heywood noted the role
of management in the limited success of the effort to get miners tested so that those

who could benefit from ART could be identified. But he was also deeply critical of the failure of the mine union to confront HIV and to provide the dynamic moral and public health leadership needed to mobilize and educate its members.

> The National Union of Mineworkers (NUM) has been absolutely hopeless on AIDS. There's a kind of macho culture in the mining industry. A lot of them are migrant workers. There's a lot of superstition and custom amongst people. So dealing with HIV requires much more than dealing with HIV. It means dealing with people's beliefs and ancestors and witchcraft and nonpathogenic causes of illness; and the union just wasn't up to it. Strangely enough, it goes right back to the beginning of this epidemic where, in the late 1980s, they suppressed some research that was done on mine workers' sexual behavior, because it showed large numbers of mine workers having sex with other mine workers and also a large number of mine workers having sex with sex workers. I've engaged the NUM for years on issues of HIV, but whilst they make the right noises in the national office, it doesn't get down to the people who work "at the coal face."
> So even those people who do go on to treatment do so as individuals, without telling the person that they live in a bunk next to in a hostel or that they work next to, that "I'm on antiretroviral treatment. I've got AIDS." So even in the mines, despite theoretical access to treatment, you've got 3,000 people being terminated for medical reasons per annum, and most of them die within six months. They work till they're so sick that they can't work any longer; then they get repatriated to rural areas of the Transkei and so on—well, Lusikisiki is the exception—all the areas around where there's nothing, not antiretrovirals, not other drugs, not palliative care, and they're gone.

After 2002, even as he pressed for an accelerated expansion of ART for miners, Brink increasingly turned to what was missing from his HIV program: HIV care, including ART, for the miners' dependents and those who had been compelled to leave mine employment. He introduced flexibility into the program, so that workers' dependents could receive testing and counseling services and miners' retrenchment packages could include a limited period of ART. More ambitious still was Brink's effort to find mechanisms to support the testing and treatment of whole communities, doing so by developing partnerships with localities and nongovernmental organizations and by seeking international funding to support Anglo American's efforts.

> Unless we get to absolutely everybody—contacts, dependents, multiple spouses—we're not going to deal with the epidemic. I've always said we can never do it on our own; we have to go beyond the workplace. We will go

beyond our business and go back to the community, and we will look at community health issues. We'll identify what the priority issues are, and we will start making a contribution to dealing with these issues. They may be lack of access to water or basic primary health care services. We simply said, "Let's identify six communities associated with our operations in South Africa," and we're actually putting resources and expertise in making sure it all happens.

Ultimately, we want primary health care clinics in those communities functioning effectively, AIDS-aware, friendly to young people and to people who are HIV positive. That provides a platform from which you can then provide antiretroviral therapy. And that's the next step.

In seeking communities linked historically to mining, the Eastern Cape's Transkei region was an obvious choice. In 2003, when Nelson Mandela visited the Lusikisiki area, Brink arranged for the former president to see AngloGold's clinic there, inviting a three-way partnership among his company, the Mandela Foundation, and Médecins sans Frontières.

Down in Lusikisiki, MSF has got a pilot project for providing antiretroviral therapy. Our associate, AngloGold, has a primary health care clinic in the town of Lusikisiki which is a pristine building and very nicely set up, but not that many patients. And close by, within a kilometer, is the government's village clinic, which is a set of containers. They see 300 patients a day in those containers without running water; the contrast between these is ridiculous. And we've been aware of it and wanting to do something. Nelson Mandela was going down to Lusikisiki to launch the MSF program and to administer the first dose of treatment to the first selected patient. But we organized that he would come to visit the AngloGold clinic, and it was somewhat embarrassing, because there were no patients there. And I'm sure he knew exactly what this was all about. And, you know, he was basically saying, "Go on, let's make this happen. We've got to get better use of this."

In 2005, the village clinic moved into AngloGold's facility.

Yet, despite its power, wealth, and access to foreign financial sources, Anglo American's ability to transform AIDS treatment in South Africa was limited. It could not take on the tasks that only government can, something Brink made quite clear in 2004.

It can only be sustainable if government actually pays for it, and that's the way it's got to be. I think government's going to resist. There are signs that it's cracking a bit and they're going to change, but if government won't come to the party, we will go to the international donors and say, "You come in, help us kick it off; let us get it off the ground." I am absolutely convinced within a few years, government will be paying for ART. We need bridging finance, just to show that we can do it. It can be done in a responsible way, and it will have an enormous impact on behavior and attitudes to HIV if we get this going. We have already made application to PEPFAR, the President's Emergency Plan for AIDS Relief, the U.S. government–initiated program. They want 2 million people on antiretroviral therapy by 2005. We'd like to be part of that. And for me, that's a much more sustainable solution than having a policy that says we'll provide for some dependents, the lucky ones.

But he remained painfully aware of the depths of ambivalence that still characterized the government's response.

I sat in meetings with the minister of health, and I can just picture her sitting there and saying, "We will treat all the opportunistic infections. I will legislate to make sure that they treat every single person that comes in sick with TB or meningitis or whatever it is; we will treat these opportunistic infections." And I wanted to say to her, "Of course, we must treat the opportunistic infections, but unless we also treat the underlying immune deficiency, it will be an incredible waste of money. The priority is not the opportunistic diseases; the priority is to tackle the root cause of the problem, to restore the immune system by killing the HIV. Let's treat them with ART."

As a doctor and manager, Brink's response to the government's failure to act remained one of outrage and dismay.

This is a source of constant amazement today, that we can still watch people die and deny them access to treatment. It's just bizarre. We still measure blood pressures and we put people on expensive medication for hypertension on the off chance that in 30 years' time we might save them from having a stroke. Yet you can have somebody right here who you know is going to die in a year's time without access to treatment, and we say, "Well, you can't have that." And there's no earthly reason! The cost is probably similar. It is just too fickle to fathom.

The Limits of Piecemeal Change

Those who worked in the public sector hospitals also struggled to overcome the constraints imposed by the national government's policy. Driven by the desire to do more, they sought out funding opportunities, both domestic and international.

While some were successful, for others such efforts met with frustration that only served to underscore the limits of approaches that attempted to circumvent the intransigence of a government that would not fund access to treatment.

Paul Kocheleff, who knew from a life's work in Africa how resources limited what he could do as a physician, was haunted by the feeling that despite his efforts at Grey's and Edendale hospitals in Pietermaritzburg, he was "hunting dinosaurs with a water gun, especially when we looked at the result of giving antiretroviral drugs in other countries." The remarkable response of the few patients at his clinic who could afford to buy medicine only intensified his sense of frustration. In December 2002, he was informed that there was a very good prospect that if he submitted a proposal to the Nelson Mandela Fund, he would be able to obtain support for the treatment of several hundred patients with antiretrovirals. In fact, he believed that he would be providing treatment within weeks. In the end, at a meeting where he anticipated receiving the award, he was told that the grant would go elsewhere.

> We had got the help, free of charge, from three pharmacists in town here
> and in a rural area 20 kilometers from here. And all the people from
> that area would be put on antiretroviral drugs in that project, would get
> properly the medication, and we had organized monitoring. So we were
> really devastated and not understanding why somebody who made such a
> lot of pressure to get a proposal, even asking the private pharmacists to
> come to the meeting, would say, "First, we don't have this big amount of
> money. We have only a small amount. The big amount maybe will come
> later, and that small amount we have decided to give to another province."

Adding to the sting of the unanticipated rejection was the recognition that patients would have to be told.

> We were so sure that this time we would have money to buy antiretroviral
> drugs that we made a selection among the patients. And they were told,
> "You know, this time you will get the antiretroviral drugs. Just wait, we will
> contact you." And so we had to tell the patients the next time, "We
> have nothing," and that was the worst of the aspects. For the patient,
> that was very, very difficult. I'm afraid that Africans are used to bad news,
> and so they said, "Oh."

For Umesh Lalloo, head of the Department of Medicine at the Nelson R. Mandela School of Medicine in Durban, the possibility that the UN-sponsored Global Fund to Fight AIDS, Tuberculosis and Malaria could underwrite the provision of antiretrovirals in some urban and rural hospitals and clinics in KwaZulu-Natal led to the preparation of a complex and ambitious request for support. On learning of his submission, the minister of health, Tshabalala-Msimang, was outraged.[34] The provincial Department of Health, acting at the behest of the minister, instructed him to withdraw the application, a request which he initially ignored. In the end, the Global Fund approved his proposal. At that juncture, the national government charged him with having failed to obey its orders. Told to relinquish the award, he refused. In the following year, Lalloo, who had responded to the intimidation of apartheid by actively fighting against it, was subjected to increasing political pressure.

> We were advised that this had gone to the level of the state president's office. Ours was seen as a plan to sabotage what government was planning to do, and so at that level you already felt very uncomfortable. And all the meetings we had with government officials didn't help to allay that anxiety at all. One felt intimidated and when one is warned by senior, high-ranking people that you'd better be careful—whether it had any basis, I don't know—but I certainly felt very intimidated. There were times when I felt like I should just leave the country and work elsewhere. I was worried about my family, although there were not direct threats. I just felt worried.

Finally, Lalloo capitulated to the demand that the provincial authorities be given control over the grant. "Ultimately I took the decision to relent in allowing the provincial Department of Health to control the grant, if it meant that by us digging in our heels, we'd lose the grant altogether. We would have liked not to have to [make] that choice."

It was against a backdrop of corporate innovations in the private sector and small-scale, although important, achievements in providing antiretroviral treatment in the public health care system, made possible by the support of international organizations, that mounting pressure, skillfully spearheaded by the Treatment Action Campaign, was put on the government of Thabo Mbeki. For those who had begun to witness the effects of antiretrovirals on the sick and dying, the barriers erected by the government were increasingly seen as medically and morally indefensible. Deep division within the South African ruling coalition—the South African Communist Party and the Congress of South African Trade Unions opposed the ANC position on ART—eroded the government's capacity to hold firm against global opinion and pressure from the popular alliances that had been formed in the struggle for treatment access. By mid-2003, the government was compelled to do what it had so tenaciously resisted since the late 1990s. It formally acknowledged the right of those infected with HIV to effective antiretroviral treatment.

6

New Beginnings?

The Wall Comes Down

> It was a huge march, a total cross-section, a visible number of doctors and
> nurses, a large religious and trade union presence, a lot of just ordinary
> people. Fifty percent of the people we brought from Johannesburg had
> HIV. It was an incredibly moving experience. A lot of people who went on
> the march died in the months following.

So recalled Mark Heywood, describing a demonstration demanding access to
antiretroviral therapy organized by the Treatment Action Campaign in Cape Town
on February 14, 2003. The importance of the march for people with HIV was
captured by Hermann Reuter, who headed MSF's clinical effort in Lusikisiki.

> We organized a bus from here, 65 people, to join that march. And that
> was, for most people, their first time out of Lusikisiki. So it was an expe-
> rience to go to that march and see a march with so many people. And
> there was a child—she was a patient from Khayelitsha—she spoke about
> being raped by her uncle and being HIV positive, and her stepfamily
> was waiting for her to die. And then she started antiretroviral treatment,
> and now the family wants her to become a lawyer. They heard these
> stories from the horse's mouth. They came back so enthusiastic, and they
> educated the community about HIV testing.

That TAC would use the occasion of Thabo Mbeki's state-of-the-nation address to
stage its protest before Parliament "caused great anger within the ANC," said
Heywood. "It made them very, very pissed off."

The ANC's bitterness was only intensified when, in the next month, TAC
launched its Dying for Treatment campaign, which involved acts of civil disobedience and charges that the minister of health was guilty of "culpable homicide."[1]

That the campaign began just before Sharpeville Day, which memorializes the March 21, 1960, massacre of anti-apartheid demonstrators by the South African police, only served to deepen the gulf. "We and hundreds of others are participating in civil disobedience because millions of people with HIV/AIDS in our country are dying premature and avoidable deaths."[2] As he wrote to justify TAC's decision, Zackie Achmat, the movement's chairperson, declared:

> After countless attempts at talking, public pressure and even a court case, the government allows the deaths to continue. . . . Politeness disguises the moral and legal culpability of the politicians. We believe that the personal crises faced by many of our families, friends, nurses, doctors, colleagues and their children should be turned into discomfort and a crisis for the politicians and bureaucrats who continue to deny our people medicine.[3]

The political and ideological complexity of the decision to engage in civil disobedience was captured by the ways in which the government and the powerful Congress of South African Trade Unions (COSATU), an ally of the ANC which had come to support TAC, sought to characterize the effort. It was a battle over the symbolic heart of post-apartheid South Africa. For the national executive committee of the ANC, TAC had done nothing less than betray the legacy of the struggle against the old regime. Its "unlawful actions would undercut the institutions of democracy for which so many South Africans have fought and made sacrifices." COSATU, on the other hand, sought to make clear that, in joining TAC, it was not protesting against an "illegitimate government, but the government's illegitimate policies related to AIDS."[4]

Mark Heywood understood only too well the very treacherous political terrain on which TAC now found itself: "The civil disobedience campaign had me personally worried about whether it was the correct thing to do, to accuse ministers of culpable homicide and to go hard up against them, because of the danger of shutting the door permanently." But when it appeared that, in the wake of the protests, negotiations for a treatment plan were possible, and TAC suspended its civil disobedience, it was the rank and file who felt bitter and betrayed. Heywood recalled, "People were so angry and felt that we'd sold them out. I remember one person who said, 'You can suspend civil disobedience, but you can't suspend the fact that I'm dying. You can't suspend the fact that I'm in pain.'"

By mid-2003, Deputy President Jacob Zuma announced that the decision to introduce an antiretroviral treatment plan would be made as soon as possible.[5] In July, TAC was able to leak a government report that suggested that a national treatment program was, in fact, affordable.[6] And in August, the government announced that it would commit itself to the provision of treatment to the vast numbers for whom ART was a matter of life and death.

The Rollout: Who Shall Treat?

Only in mid-November was an official plan released that provided some detail on how the scaling up of the treatment would occur. Although the plan assumed that 400,000 people would develop AIDS-defining illnesses in 2004, it projected that ART would be made available to 53,000 patients in 2003–2004. In the program's second year, the cumulative number receiving antiretrovirals was to rise to 188,000. Only by 2008–2009 would the program reach its target of just under 1.5 million treated cases.[7] Inevitably, then, given the pace of the rollout, many clinics and hospitals caring for very sick children and adults would have no alternative but to wait months or years to offer therapy.

For those in facilities that were scheduled to provide ART early on, there was palpable anticipation. Caroline Armstrong recalled speaking with patients at Grey's Hospital, telling them that the rollout would begin. "We got so excited." Recalling the disappointment they had endured when a hoped-for foundation-supported effort had fallen through, those in her clinic pressured her, asking, "Is it going to happen, or is it just talk?" Reassuringly, she replied, "No, it's going to happen. There's been too much pressure on the government for it not to happen, and they've given their word it's going to happen. When, we don't know." Others were far more skeptical, given the hostility that the health authorities had evinced all along. Especially dubious about when the drugs would arrive, Paul Nijs at Edendale Hospital, said, "Until they are on my desk, I will not believe this." And to protect his patients, he refused to talk about when that might be.

> I try not to tell my patients, because I don't know. I will mark on my diary the names of the patients. I will put "this is a good candidate," but I will not tell him, because what if it never happens? Some of these patients are in an advanced stage of the disease. Some might have an infection or a disease, and they will not overcome it. I don't want to tell them.

For clinicians not identified as being part of the initial phase, the experience could be shattering. Helga Holst, whose efforts at McCord Hospital in Durban had won international attention, had every reason to believe that her institution would be selected, based on its expertise and because, as a private institution, it had no alternative but to charge patients for treatment. At a meeting with a senior provincial health official, she was told:

> McCord would not be considered because we were so far ahead of the game and because of the issue of equity. We wouldn't be getting any assistance or help towards our AIDS work and programs until the rest of the province had been brought up to the same standard we were currently

providing. It was like the carpet was taken from under my feet. I was really disappointed; it really hurt.

For Holst's patients, who had limited resources, the decision was also a deep blow.

> We have always been encouraging patients that sooner or later the De-
> partment of Health, the government, will see the light. There has been talk
> of universal rollout, so we said, "Please hang on," month by month by
> month. So we kept telling our patients, "See how much you can scrounge
> to get the money to pay for this month's antiretrovirals."

Holst noted that some knew that they would have to interrupt their treatment because they could not afford to continue. Given her religious faith, her commitment, and the support her efforts had received from both within South Africa and internationally, Holst declared, in the face of the government's decision, "There is no way I'm going to sit down and say, 'No, I'm not interested in going any further.'"

The story for Bernhard Gaede was very different. His hospital, too, was not selected for the initial rollout. But, with rural Emmaus understaffed and overextended, he felt relieved of a potential new burden. In February 2004, he wrote in a letter:

> We are hardly coping to see the outpatients that come every day. We
> cannot manage the antenatal high-risk patients. We've stopped going to the
> primary health clinics in the area. All ambulances with emergencies have
> been diverted to another hospital to decrease the load on us. In the crisis we
> now face, ART is a pipe dream.

Yet, deeply moved by the plight of his patients, he also acknowledged that he became despondent when he would "sit in the outpatients' department and see young, emaciated people with AIDS losing hope." And so, despite the sense of "relief" he felt at not being asked to take on an ART service, he confessed, "It feels strange to see the new possibilities so close ... and yet have so far to go."

Waiting for ART

Whatever enthusiasm was unleashed with the publication of the government's rollout plan was quickly dampened by frustration as delays followed delays. Despite the number of people dying of AIDS, estimated by TAC at 800 a day, the government appeared to be responding with characteristic truculence. In January 2004, MSF's Eric Goemaere noted that, despite the changes occurring on the provincial level, the national effort seemed all but frozen. "I don't see what's happening at the moment. There is hardly any progress. Here is an army of good will that is literally jumping to its feet, but someone forgot the ammunition, and there is no way we can go forward without that." At Johannesburg Hospital, Dalu Ndiweni appeared resigned as he said, in early 2004:

We have the feeling that it will eventually start. There are many things that need to be sorted out. You learn to take what politicians say—until it is set, you can't be absolutely sure. Initially, when ART was announced, we thought we would have started by now. Unfortunately, the medications have not come through.

Indeed, it was not until early 2004, five months after the release of its plan, that the government, placed under enormous pressure by TAC and approaching national elections, agreed to speed the process for purchasing the needed drugs.

The exacting, bureaucratic investigation of clinics to document and approve their readiness to provide treatment also slowed the rollout. Ashraf Grimwood, who had been a public health officer in Cape Town early in his career and then went on to private practice, had served on the committee that prepared the rollout plan. He could only express dismay over a process that had squandered the hopes of August 2003.

The work-up to the plan, getting it all done, was so amazing. We just thought it was too good to be true. You felt that we were on the brink of a major, major revolution in this country in the sense of taking the bull by the horns and saying, "Let's do it." Now you end up in bureaucratic nonsense. "We can't do that. The pharmacy's not the right size. We don't have enough fridges. We don't have enough space." This is bullshit; there are people dying out there.

Commenting on the state of affairs, the *Mail and Guardian* wrote:

Here we are two months into 2004, and we are singing the same tune we have since 1999; our government exercises absolutely no leadership in the fight against HIV/AIDS; every inch of progress (and it must be mea-sured in torturous inches) has been won in street battles, propaganda wars and the courts. . . . The lack of progress in the AIDS war is clearly neither financial nor intellectual, nor is it about capacity. It is about absence of political will at the center.[8]

But despite the impediments, the provision of antiretroviral treatment in the public sector did begin, first on a large scale in the Western Cape and then in Gauteng, the economic hub of South Africa, because provincial health officials there were committed to providing ART. Where such officials remained reluctant, however, the experience was very different. Eula Mothibi, who had been involved in the establishment of a successful clinic in Cape Town supported by the Nelson Mandela Fund, had been repeatedly implored by the coordinator for HIV programs in the vast Northern Cape Province to "Come home, come home." Mothibi decided to accept the challenge of the rollout to serve "her people." Kimberley was to be the coordinating site for about 12 towns, the farthest of which was a five-hour drive. Other regional centers would function in a similar way. But when she arrived at Kimberley Hospital, the center of her operations for the entire province, she found only "a little office." In 2004 she reported, "I don't even have a phone. I haven't gotten a fax machine either, and I haven't gotten a computer." It was only her relationship to the people and the community that kept her from returning to Cape Town. "A lot of people are people I know. I know their relatives, I know their families; they know my family."

Drugs into Bodies: Urgency in a Resource-Poor Environment

Within clinical settings, the speed with which efforts were made to increase the number of patients getting antiretroviral therapy depended on the extent of hospitals' cooperation, the resources made available to treatment services, and, most strikingly, the devotion and commitment of the doctors and nurses involved.

Because of a number of factors—including the Mandela Children's Foundation funds, the continued decrease in the cost of the antiretroviral drugs, and the promise of antiretrovirals in the public health sector, to which MSF patients in Lusikisiki could eventually be transferred—Hermann Reuter was able to provide ART to as many patients as came forward and required it.

> Choosing who would be first to be put on ART was no issue at all. We had a big budget. Initially, ART was very expensive, and you had a budget for 30 patients, for 50 patients. In Khayelitsha, we were lucky, 180 patients. And then you had to ration and say, "Which 180 patients do I choose?" But in Lusikisiki, from the beginning, we said, "All patients." We had enough budget. ART was cheaper. We had enough confidence that after two or three years we would be able to hand patients over to the government. We also realized that the longer you wait to put somebody on ART, the more difficult it gets. So we decided, when people need ART, they get it. We don't wait.

Over the following year, the MSF clinics were able to swiftly enroll patients who met the national eligibility criteria for treatment and possessed the ability to come to a clinic, a willingness to disclose their HIV status to a treatment partner, and the perceived ability to adhere to therapy. At the end of 2003, 12 people were in treatment. Twelve months later, that number had grown to 551. Reuter's success was an answer to those, especially in the national government, who were skeptical about whether ART could be used outside South Africa's metropolitan areas. His experience was also atypical.

Linda-Gail Bekker, whose own service in Guguletu on the outskirts of Cape Town was funded by the international Global Fund to Fight AIDS, Tuberculosis and Malaria, gave voice to the challenges facing even the most ardent in their desire to expand treatment. With 500 patients receiving ART in early 2005 and 80 more per month being screened for eligibility, she noted:

> The main goal is really to get the numbers up, so that we don't have large numbers of people waiting and possibly dying while waiting to get onto treatment. One can try and have everything perfect to get people onto treatment, but there's a significant death rate whilst one does that. One has to eventually weigh up the risk-and-benefit ratio of whether you'd rather get them onto treatment or sort out problems, but you've got to get that ratio just right.

Having been accredited to provide antiretrovirals in February 2004, Tony Moll's Church of Scotland Hospital was among the very first in KwaZulu-Natal to begin the provision of medication under the government's rollout.

> We were very excited, and immediately things started changing. We started putting things into place to be able to give antiretrovirals on a much wider scale. We prepared a group of nine patients very quickly, getting the CD4 counts ready and meeting entrance criteria. March 24, 2004, we announced, was going to be the day that we would actually give out antiretroviral therapy.

The debut was marked by the thrill of a new beginning and the inevitable political trappings such an event was bound to call forth.

> An official from the provincial Department of Health joined us that day. That was our launch. The BBC was also there, and they covered it. Actually, a few hours after everything had happened and our party was over and the people had gone home, I got a very serious telephone call from people from the Department of Health, saying, "Whatever you do, no newspapers, no TV. BBC, tell them to block all the information." And the scare was that we had run ahead in KwaZulu-Natal. The national minister hadn't yet officially said we're starting with the rollout! So they told me, "Just tell everybody to shut up now." So I phoned the BBC, and I said, "We can only say that we've done it once the minister of health nationally says, 'Go ahead.'" But there were nine patients who received medication, and it was a very happy day for us. The patients, their families were with us; the nurses were with us; people from our district office were there.

Once the program began, Moll and his colleagues, sensing renewed possibilities and deep urgency, surged ahead. In nine months, he, his small nursing staff, and two counselors brought 360 patients into treatment.

After those nine, things moved very fast. The government told us, "Don't worry. Whatever you order in terms of medication, we will be able to supply you." So it wasn't the medication that was a problem, and it wasn't the laboratory facilities; they were ready to receive as many CD4s as we sent them. What was particularly burdensome was that we were one of only four hospitals chosen in the province. So we had people coming from really far, hearing announcements on the radio that these are the four hospitals that are on board. And we had people coming from Durban, from Dundee, from Newcastle, from Johannesburg, coming to us. The clientele built up quite a lot. Very close hospitals were starting to send buses full of patients on a weekly basis to us.

What very soon became our ceiling was our own hands and our own small group of staff members. And they were incredible. On the days they were on duty, they were prepared to work through the night. But for me, it was different, because I'm on duty every day. I had this conflict in myself that, if I worked a little harder, I could help a couple more people, and if I worked on a Saturday morning, I could help even more people. In the end, I could see that I was just becoming chronically tired, and I wasn't doing my work properly. I was taking shortcuts where I shouldn't be taking shortcuts. I spoke to people and said, "You know, we could do so many more people, but we're short of staff." And even the provincial people said, "Well, Tony, then what you must do is do what you can do." That helped me to see that it was more important to have a service that was running well and run properly, where the wheel wasn't going to come off. So we just said, "OK, we'll work extra hours, but we'll stop at that time."

Serving as an additional restraint on Moll's efforts, as well as those in other hospitals, was the discovery that placing large numbers of patients on ART could have unanticipated but, in retrospect, predictable consequences for those responsible for managing the hospital's wards.

What started happening was one or two patients came in with side effects and needed to be admitted to hospital. And these junior doctors were in charge of the wards, and they found themselves responsible for somebody who was on ART, and they themselves weren't confident in managing this. Quite correctly, they came back to me and said, "Now, put the brakes on." What we did was, we brought them up to date, and they felt, "OK, now we know when to admit; this is when to stop treatment." So we had actually run ahead of ourselves a little bit.

It was months after the adult service began to provide antiretroviral treatment that the Department of Pediatrics was given approval to provide drugs to children. Like his colleague Tony Moll, François Eksteen, who had for so long watched his patients suffer and die, approached this opportunity with zeal. Time, Eksteen knew, was not his ally, and waiting lists for very sick children were morally unacceptable to him.

Waiting lists can go on into two months or even longer. I just feel it's a potentially fatal disease, a disease that potentially can cause severe suffering. I've got some children whose CD4s are very low, and I just feel one cannot wait with that. So I just personally feel that we must start as soon as possible.

Early on, Moll discovered how single-minded his colleague could be.

One evening, I came into his clinic, and I found the lights still on and the staff still there and François was working. And the whole waiting room was full of children with their mothers, waiting. It was after 8:00 at night! It was dark outside; the public transport would have stopped by then. So I said, "You know, you're not going to finish. You're going to be working till 2:00 tonight if you really see everybody that's in the waiting room. Those patients who are on therapy or who are here for follow-up, finish them tonight. And those who are new patients, let them sleep over, and we will sort them out in the morning." François is right now feeling that exhilaration that I felt with the rollout, that now suddenly the children are coming in big numbers, and he is facing his own limitations in helping them.

In Pietermaritzburg, Paul Kocheleff had also waited—sometimes buoyed by hope, on other occasions despairing—for the moment when he could provide his patients at Grey's Hospital with antiretrovirals. Four months after Tony Moll had begun, Kocheleff believed that he done everything to make his start-up smooth, but things turned out very differently. His clinic would be dogged by the same dearth of professional staff that other locales would experience, and his ambitious plans to treat the 900 patients who qualified for ART would be thwarted by the mundane limits of a public hospital.

Our idea was that probably we can start with 10 patients a day, working five days a week. That means 50 patients per week, 200 per month. We expected that in four months, five months, everybody would be on treatment. And then we had the meeting with the pharmacy, and they had a totally different opinion about the program. They wanted to have 5 patients per week! That means it will take years to reach 900! And the discussion was a bit hard, but finally we agreed that maybe we can try and see what happens. So we had to slow down a little bit. But after a few weeks, we were able to increase the number of patients starting. At the moment, it's between 100 and 150 per month, so it's not far from what we wanted at the start.

By January 2005, he had enrolled 700 patients.

Even when faced with less than enthusiastic hospital administrators, those who believed that they had no alternative but to overcome obstacles were able to achieve remarkable feats. At Baragwanath Hospital, 51-year-old Alan Karstaedt, who oversees the adult HIV clinic, had been able to put 1,500 patients on treatment in the six months following the commencement of ART in April 2004.

It's been really rough, with very long hours. Sometimes the clinics have finished at 7:30 at night. We've got more doctors now, but we've had at various times only three or four. We just committed ourselves to getting as many people on treatment as quickly as possible. We've had to cut corners.

Karstaedt, who had rejected applying for promotions to more administrative positions because "clinical work is what I love and enjoy," had taken great pride in the fact that, over the years, he had been able to spend time speaking with his patients, resisting the pressure to "just turn them into faceless ciphers." But he had to acknowledge that his commitment to providing ART now compelled him to make compromises.

Basically you're trading off, getting more people onto treatment and more people hopefully surviving longer and living independent, quality lives versus that other form of clinical interaction and satisfaction. But given the number of patients who are going to need to be put on treatment, I think this will become the model, whether it's ideal or not.

Like Karstaedt, Tammy Meyers's efforts to forge a treatment program for children with AIDS were affected by the enormous burdens and budgetary limits shouldered by the administration at Baragwanath Hospital.

HIV is not business as usual. I think the hospital administration, the Pediatrics Department, even the Medicine Department in this hospital feel that HIV is one of the many things that they have to deal with. Which is understandable. It's a huge hospital, it's almost like a beast to manage, and there was a huge budget deficit at the end of 2003. So the whole administration was changed. The main goal was to make sure that they could deal with the budget deficit.

As a consequence, her drive and enthusiasm were blocked by obstacles that had become all too familiar to her over the years. Although she had been able, by early 2005, to enroll 400 patients in what she thought might be the largest children's treatment program in the country, she was still far short of the 1,000 patients who she believed needed care.

> We were down to two doctors at one stage, just after the rollout started. It was incredible to know that you've got the treatment and that you could be actually providing it to those who need it. I think it was more traumatic than before, because *we* were now the rate-limiting factor, and it was very hard to deal with that. So we fought as much as we could, fought with the hospital administration. There were people in the Department of Health who actually wanted this program to succeed; so we tried to push as much as possible and managed to get some extra posts and employ more doctors.

Although not formally part of the government's rollout, the ART program at McCord Hospital represented a significant locus of care. Helga Holst remained true to her word that she would not be defeated. She recalled, "We took the challenge and said, 'If we're not going to get help from the government, we're going to do it on our own.'" As of January 2004, McCord was treating about 600 patients who were covered by medical insurance, paying out of pocket, or had the support of their families or employers. Partnering with an American-based foundation, McCord successfully applied for support from the U.S. government's President's Emergency Plan for AIDS Relief (PEPFAR). The award would cover the 600 patients, eliminating their need to pay expenses; a supplement increased that number to 900. "It was just such an awesome thing for us. It has reaffirmed my faith at a much deeper level. Not that I didn't believe God could answer prayers. I just didn't know quite how He was going to manage this one. It seemed almost too big."

Recognizing that even this expanded effort merely began to meet the needs of people with HIV, McCord sought additional support to enlarge its treatment capacity. With waiting lists stretching months into the future, there was a moral imperative to do so. When the anticipated funding failed to materialize, the consequences were devastating to the staff and to patients preparing to begin treatment. Jane Hampton, who had reveled in not having to raise the issue of drug costs with her patients, as she had had to do in the past, described the pain she felt on hearing this disappointing news.

> I woke with a very heavy heart—a day when we would have to pass very difficult news on to people who would probably have woken with excitement in their hearts—hopeful that at last the day had dawned when they could start their ART. Those arriving for their third sessions of training, who had had preparatory blood tests, and investigations to

exclude TB and a clinical consultation the week before, and had been assured that there was no medical or social reason not to start ART, would have to be told that today is not the day. The majority had no possibility of self-funding. One person had just returned from her nearest rollout site, having been given a date to return six months later.

Ultimately, some additional funding was obtained, permitting McCord to enlarge its rolls by another 250 patients. This was not the target it had set. But it was enough to meet the needs of those who had been prepared to start care and who had suffered such a disappointing setback. But that expansion had other consequences. With a hint of irony, Holst described the "AIDS envy" that set in at that time, affecting those not engaged in the hospital's AIDS commitment. The success of the HIV program, she said,

> allowed us as a hospital to take a bit of the focus away from the AIDS work, which has been the big complaint amongst the staff not involved with AIDS. They said, "We're becoming an AIDS hospital. That's all that people are talking about, and it's the only thing where the publicity comes. What about our work? Isn't what we're doing important? Isn't that also important?"

The experiences of those who had participated in the first stages of the rollout could serve to bolster and encourage those who had yet to begin. Bernhard Gaede, who had expressed such despair because he seemed to be mired in a failing institution that could barely meet the most basic needs of its patients and who had experienced subsequent relief at being passed over for the initial rollout, found the courage to seek accreditation for an ART program after visiting Tony Moll.

> The first task was to get over the hurdle of wondering whether we would be able to do it or not. In the first meetings, our people were very skeptical. When we looked at the manuals, it felt like we don't have all of that, we can't do it, we can't jump over that hurdle, it's too big. And then we visited Tony Moll at the Church of Scotland Hospital; hordes of people milling about the clinic and being tested in this more or less organized chaos, and people being quite open about it. I think that was quite a strong motivator. On the way back in the car, the staff were saying, "Well, Tony says, 'Just do it. You must just set it up; you can do it; just go and do it.'" And that was really inspirational for some of the nurses and also one of the other doctors who came with us. She was saying, "They get adherence of 90–95 percent, so why can't we?"

With a newfound sense of the possibilities, Gaede and his staff began to prepare their application to the Department of Health.

We needed to get protocols for how the service would run, for the different stages of the service. We needed to make sure that the lab services were in place, that the pharmacy followed the requirements. Do we have the space? Do we have the staff, and do the various people know what they should be doing? Do we have protocols for the different treatments? We had to have a conceptual understanding of where would patients come from, how would they get to Emmaus, how would they be followed up, how would they be supported? We drew a conceptual diagram, and that motivated people quite a lot, saying, "Yes, this is something that we can do."

On December 10, 2004, the hospital received its accreditation to provide ART. "For the team here," said Gaede, "it was just complete elation." Within one and a half years, 15 people per week were being brought into treatment. On May 10, 2006, Emmaus enrolled its 500th patient.

Drugs into Bodies: Institutional Inertia

If a mix of administrative support, resources, and clinician enthusiasm could shape the response of those who grasped at the opportunity to provide ART, its absence could serve to retard the extension of treatment. Although the rollout had officially begun at Johannesburg Hospital in April 2004, Dalu Ndiweni reported that, nine months later, about 130 children were receiving treatment. The hospital had poorly prepared for the provision of antiretrovirals, in part because of the ongoing burdens of caring for children with AIDS.

We're literally sinking under the load of clinical problems, opportunistic infections that are HIV-related, or AIDS-related illnesses inside the ward. We're just grappling with putting in the drip, rehydrating somebody, treating the pneumonia, treating the PCP, treating the TB and things like that, without saying, "Look here, how do we get ourselves ready to move on?"

Eula Mothibi remained thwarted and frustrated, having been given virtually none of the resources she needed to execute a rollout in the Northern Cape, the country's largest province. For six months, as she tried to start her ART service at Kimberley Hospital, she had been the only doctor. She had pleaded for additional support: "We've got almost a three-month waiting list because I am alone. We can barely cope with that many." Because she was able to add only eight patients a week, the list kept growing. "I can't get through to people who are managing these things," she reported. "I'm struggling."

Among the most striking examples of how administrative attitudes, resources, and clinician concerns could conspire to slow the pace of bringing people into treatment was the situation that prevailed at South Africa's second largest hospital, King Edward VIII Hospital. Kogie Naidoo, speaking about the adult HIV clinic, believed that provincial authorities had not supported a rapid rollout at King Edward VIII because it was a sophisticated tertiary care facility. The administration of the hospital was also less than engaged.

> [The provincial health officials'] primary goal was to start off the rollout at facilities that could not give secondary or tertiary level care, to really target community hospitals, district-level hospitals, so the development of infrastructure, the staffing and other resources, was upgraded at district-level hospitals first. The other problem was that there wasn't sufficient will among the management of the hospital to get going. It wasn't recognized that this was their priority; it was quite easy to overlook what needed to be done and focus on other things.

Raziya Bobat, also at King Edward VIII, lamented the state of affairs in the Pediatric Department. Although she believed that as many as 300 clinic patients could benefit from ART, less than 80 children were receiving such care in January 2005.

> It's frustrating. The numbers we are treating are so small, and that's because we don't have enough human resources. That's the reality. It's going very slowly. We would love to be able to say we can put all our kids on treatment right now. Apart from the human resources being one of the factors that determine how quickly we can treat, we're very strict about the mum going through all the steps that we have set down. So it's social worker, adherence counselor, back to social worker, back to adherence counselor; and the social workers have come up with so many problems and so many issues that have to be addressed before you can actually begin.

She revealed a sense of resignation as she noted that her clinic had a three-month waiting list. "Well, three months is not too bad in our opinion right now, because, with our specialist clinics, we always have bookings waiting for three months, six months. It's not too bad."

The adult HIV clinic at King Edward was the responsibility of Yunus Moosa, a doctor who had recently returned from training in infectious disease in the United States, where he had earned a Ph.D. He believed that it would be a grave mistake for him to be involved in the hands-on provision of ART to AIDS patients.

> When I got here, I was told, "Well, the ART rollout is on your doorstep. You went to the States; you have qualified. You have learned how to use ART. So you are the man. You are responsible now for creating and administering and running the rollout at King Edward." But that's primary

health care! I've spent most of my life training to be a superspecialist, and now you want me to come here and practice primary health care? I cannot sit in a clinic and see patient after patient, dishing out ART. I think my role has to be bigger than that, or different from that. So I refused to be a primary care physician in an ART rollout. I'm happy to be involved in trying to set it up and administer it, but I'm certainly not going to be involved in administering it at the ground level. What I'm happy to do and need to get involved in is creating a secondary structure that would allow for complicated patients that other doctors do not know how to deal with. So I tried to set it up so that HIV is just part of my responsibility, although that's been very, very difficult. It's virtually consumed 90 percent of my time.

The doctor who was ultimately chosen to run the clinic had no experience with HIV care.

We asked the hospital manager to identify somebody, so they pulled a doctor from the Medical Outpatient Department. He knew nothing about antiretrovirals, so we started giving him the literature, telling him about the drugs, and I told him, "You phone me as many times as you like any time of the day or night. I'm available to you." So slowly over the course of six to eight months, he's learned the ropes, and he's now pretty confident.

Less than a year after the clinic began to provide antiretrovirals, there were 390 patients being treated. The doctor who had been given the task of running the clinic had resigned his post.

As they attempted to address the limits placed on them by the public health system's capacity, providers came to realize that the drugs which had been at the center of the bitter battle between treatment activists and the government of Thabo Mbeki no longer represented the most critical problem they faced in the massive effort to extend treatment to hundreds of thousands of patients. Rather, it was now necessary to move swiftly beyond doctor- (and hospital-) centered clinics in a way that did not compromise the essentials of antiretroviral treatment. Whatever role doctors would play in the future would, of necessity, be dwarfed by the roles of nurses and counselors.

Many came to believe that, once patients were stabilized, they would have to be placed in the charge of a nurse-run system, not unlike what already existed in the nation's TB program or in AngloGold's HIV model. Bernhard Gaede was not sure that solution would be so easy to implement. He worried that the burden, once shifted to nurses, would itself be more than the system could bear. It was not that nurses were incapable of doing the clinical work, if guided by treatment protocols. Rather, the number of available nurses would be the limiting factor. "There are not endless nurses. While it's easy to say that doctors are not coping, the nurses need to do it, who will the nurses offload to? They are at the moment our safety net, but that net is also at a breaking point."

It was obvious that tertiary hospital-based clinics would have to yield to those located in urban and rural primary care settings, much as they already were in MSF's Khayelitsha and Lusikisiki ventures. Paul Kocheleff in Pietermaritzburg, who had devoted years to fostering a service that would meet the psychological as well as medical needs of his patients, regretted what he saw as both necessary and inevitable. He worried most about what would happen to the quality of HIV care. "A clinic where everybody is very concerned and wants to help would be the best place for everybody to come and have a good chance to have long-term compliance. But if we look at the numbers of patients, it is an impossibility."

Provincial Rollouts: The Haves and the Have-Nots

When, in November 2003, the government had made public its antiretroviral treatment plan, it expected that almost 200,000 patients would be receiving ART by 2005. In fact, in January of that year, only about 30,000 were receiving medication in the public sector.[9] The initial plan, which embraced equity as a guiding principle, had nevertheless made clear that because of very different levels of epidemic severity and infrastructural capacity, the numbers to be brought into care would vary widely by province. In the Eastern Cape, it was expected that approximately 18,000 would be in treatment, while in neighboring KwaZulu-Natal, the number would be 75,000. In Gauteng, where Johannesburg is located, 45,000 would be in treatment. In the very poor provinces of Mpumalanga and Limpopo, 11,000 and 22,000, respectively, were to have been in care. But in each instance, the numbers projected to be in treatment fell far short in practice. With 10,000 people in treatment in Gauteng, the shortfall was 80 percent; in KwaZulu-Natal, only about 15 percent of the projected goal was achieved. The story was even worse in the very poorest of provinces, where between 1 and 2 percent of the target had been met by early 2005. A year later, in January 2006, there had been significant improvements, but the shortfall remained striking. The number of patients receiving ART had risen to just more than 110,000, still less than half of what had been promised. By mid-2006, the number in the public sector had risen to 140,000.[10]

Commenting on the torpid pace of the government's effort, especially in the poorest regions, Treatment Action Campaign's Mark Heywood said in early 2005:

We still have provinces where almost nobody is on treatment. Mpumalanga
Province has less than 200 people on treatment, as far as we know.
North West Province has islands of treatment. Limpopo Province has less
than 200 people on treatment—this despite the fact that in Limpopo
there are health facilities with absolute capacity to run this program. One

such place is Tintswalo, which is actually linked to Witwatersrand University in Johannesburg, that to this day has not been accredited to run a treatment program, so the doctors have to illicitly treat people. TAC supplies drugs now to Tintswalo, so that they can treat a limited number of people. But it's ridiculous that we have to be doing it underhandedly.

Haroon Saloojee, head of the Division of Community Pediatrics at the University of the Witwatersrand, having left his position as chief of neonatology at Baragwanath, was equally critical of the Limpopo provincial government.

I've talked with the leadership in Limpopo Province, and there have been endless battles. They were adamant that despite Tintswalo having prior experience—probably one of the best experiences in the country in a rural setting—they were adamant that the hospital would not deliver antiretrovirals. So the question then is, Why? There is also the sense of unwillingness to move; you almost feel you have to push agendas all the time, and that's certainly true in Limpopo Province, whether it is mother-to-child transmission or antiretrovirals. The premier of that province is more of a lackey of central government; he's not willing to confront issues.

Elsewhere, the rollout was erratic. In the Eastern Cape, according to Heywood, Lusikisiki was the lone bright spot.

The Eastern Cape is a mess, again largely due to political mismanagement. The only "success story" is Lusikisiki. Hermann Reuter and the TAC and MSF have transformed that village. More people are on treatment in Lusikisiki than in the whole province of Limpopo. But its long-term sustainability depends upon the health system in that province being sorted out. You can't have an island of efficiency and ethics and decency and a sea of general mismanagement and chaos.

Heywood stressed that, even in the well-to-do and organized provinces, large pockets of poverty still existed outside the cities in areas which still lacked adequate public health infrastructure or approved rollout facilities. There, people with AIDS suffered as they did in Limpopo and the Eastern Cape.

To the credit of the Gauteng provincial government, they had about 5,000 to 6,000 people on treatment in public hospitals as of the end of 2004. But even in the best provinces, like Gauteng, it's just not going out fast enough. In June 2004, I went out to an informal settlement called Orange Farm, which is a hell hole about 60 kilometers from Johannesburg where most people live in shacks, and I met with 17 people with AIDS. We took their names, together with the names of a number of other people

that we'd collected, and promised them that we would get them onto a
treatment program. Their problem was that the nearest treatment program
was at Baragwanath Hospital. They are 60 or 70 kilometers from there;
they can't afford to get there and back in a day. Once they get there,
they couldn't wait for the whole day as they have to do. We met with the
head of health in this province, a very cordial meeting. She said, "Yes,
we'll try and do this and this, we'll open an ART site"—which, seven
months later, was still not open. Of those 17 people we promised to get on
treatment, 10 are dead now.

The Persistence of Rationing

Faced with formidable institutional, material, and political constraints and a dramatically overflowing reservoir of patients requiring antiretroviral drugs, medical
staff in clinics providing ART had to confront a series of morally and clinically
compelling questions. These were not unlike those they had encountered earlier in
the epidemic. In a resource-limited milieu, who should be treated? How should
they be selected? Who should be made to wait? Even at a hospital like McCord,
with its large treatment program, the issues had to be addressed, said Helga Holst.

> There's some—I think—healthy tension between how best do you use
> the resources given to you. Do you get better results by starting patients
> on treatment that are well and have CD4 counts above a certain level? Then
> the equity issue and the justice issue come closer to the surface. Why
> should somebody who didn't have the opportunity to be on treatment
> earlier and now is very sick be refused the opportunity, granted the risk of
> success is less?

A few argued that a commitment to treating the greatest number demanded
that the sickest, or those with the weakest immune systems, make way for patients
more likely to profit from ART. In Pietermaritzburg, Paul Nijs adopted such a
stance.

> I think the first aim of an ART program is to diminish the burden of the
> AIDS catastrophe on the public health care system. So that means, in
> my opinion, that it is more fruitful and also easier to put healthy people on
> ART treatment than to try to put people on such treatment who already
> have full-blown AIDS. I'm not saying that I will refuse to put a patient who
> has major problems on treatment, but I sometimes say it is too late. It may
> sound cruel, but you must realize that if you put a very sick patient on
> treatment, you really have to follow him up very intensively. He will run
> into problems; he will develop diarrhea, vomiting, and cannot take the

drugs. If you look at the time you spend with that patient, that time you could easily put, I would say, eight to ten healthy patients on treatment. So what is the choice? Here in KwaZulu-Natal, we're talking about half a million patients who we have to reach eventually. As one of my colleagues said, "You should concentrate on fruit that you can easily pick."

Others, taking a path that had been first pursued when antiretrovirals were available only in small research projects, screened out the sickest because they felt an overwhelming need to show the skeptical or dispirited in South Africa that anti-retrovirals could make a difference. In her pediatric HIV clinic at King Edward VIII, which treated only a fraction of those who could benefit, Raziya Bobat revealed:

I must admit that one of our exclusion criteria for the early part of the rollout is patients who have got very severe complications like cardiomy-opathy and very severe encephalopathy or any other organ failure. This is simply because we want to raise everybody's morale; you treat the child and the child starts improving, and everybody can see that they're getting better. In Malawi, they were treating the very moribund patients with ART, and they were having this very high mortality rate. And that created a problem, because people were saying, "Well, you see? The drugs are toxic, and they don't work, and the patients are dying."

In contrast, at Baragwanath Hospital, Tammy Meyers, who like Bobat treated children, was guided by a professional and moral compass that required giving priority to the sickest. The rest would follow.

We started identifying who we thought were the sicker patients who we could start immediately, as treatment became available on April 1, 2004. We identified ten children who were ready, with their low CD4s and very sick, to start treatment on that day.

Her colleague Alan Karstaedt also adopted a policy of moving the sickest of his adult patients to the head of the line.

It was a fairly rough way of doing it, but if people looked reasonably well and their CD4s were in the mid- to high hundreds, they were booked on a routine list. If they had a low CD4 or looked ill, then they were seen within a week or so, or at the next available clinic. You could put someone on ART within a week or two from the time they were first referred.

But for most clinicians, with patients' lives at stake, the need to ration ART and a commitment to a basic principle of equity led to a decision to treat on a first-come, first-served basis. In Kimberley, Eula Mothibi, despite external constraints, struggled to develop what was, for her, a just access policy.

> I get called by the assessment sites. "This person's CD4 is less than 10. This person is sick." But generally, I'm not encouraging jumping the queue, because most people come late. So I think it's unfair to those who present with a CD4 of 190; now they have to give way, lose their position in the queue. They have to give way to someone who comes in very late with a low CD4.

Like Mothibi, other clinicians often adopted a policy that appeared to obviate the need to choose. In the Western Cape, Ashraf Grimwood, who directed a network of clinics jointly funded by a British charity, ARK, and the provincial government, refused to choose which patients should first receive life-sustaining drugs.

> The thing is, we're not God. We're not making those judgment calls. People who show that they'll go through the preliminary steps, the counseling, that they understand the issues—I'm going to give you a fair chance, mate, regardless of what your CD4 is, if it's 2 or 5. We've had people with CD4 counts of 2, under 2, under 1, pull back, get better, and go for it. So we can't make that judgment call. Give everybody a fair chance. If they're going to die, they're going to die in six weeks, so what are you going to lose? Probably it's about a hundred dollars.

In Durban, Yunus Moosa, the head of infectious disease at King Edward VIII Hospital, had first advocated in favor of "patients that are best salvageable, so we can prove to the people out here that ART works," but the politics of such a standard made it an unacceptable strategy.

> The question had been, if a patient walked in with a CD4 count of 5, should we give him priority over the patient who walks in with a CD4 count of 150? We felt it would become a bit of a political hot potato. How do we decide who is sick enough or too well for immediate medication? So we decided on a blanket rule: whoever walks in first and is eligible for treatment gets into the program.

But fairness exacted a toll. It was difficult for clinicians, especially those in the trenches who encountered very sick and dying patients, to abide by the rule of first-come, first-served. Eula Mothibi confessed, "I think it's a little bit unfair, but on occasion I do push a person in with a low CD4 count. I bring them in on a Tuesday, when I run a clinic for pregnant mothers." At McCord Hospital, Henry Sunpath, who had been drawn to HIV care because the emergency room in which he had worked in the 1990s had refused to hear the pleas of AIDS patients, recognized a similar moment now. "We have people coming here to us with their relatives, young sons and daughters, parents, and they say, 'Please do something.'" It was the same plea that had moved him years earlier—when he had seen the crowds of untreated patients at another hospital—that struck him so forcefully in 2005. He continued, "As a clinician, you're faced with the patient, and you want to do something for that patient, no matter how sick that patient is."

McCord developed a hybrid system of access, one that adhered to the principle of first-come, first-served, but which acknowledged the moral claims of the sickest as well. Jane Hampton described the policy that evolved in 2004.

> It's been a big change in the last year. There are always a whole lot more people that need treatment than can be treated, and so there are still people that have to wait; but now it's waiting, it's not, "Sorry, you can't afford it, so you can't have it." It's not money that's the thing that's keeping people from treatment. It's waiting lists; it's the fact that you can only cope with so many people in a particular month. When the funding first came through, we thought, people who are critically ill and can't wait, maybe we should try and see them first; and it turned out to be an absolute nightmare. You had to have very clear guidelines of who you should fast-track and who you shouldn't. At the moment, we've got a very limited fast track, people that have actually been admitted to hospital and are on the wards, so they're already under care and already have been seen and worked up. One day out of the five, we have a clinic for them, so they don't have to wait at the end of the queue. But for everyone else, there's just a queue system, first-come, first-served.

Monitoring Patients' Lives

The extension of antiretroviral therapy, the transformation of people with HIV into patients under lifelong treatment, inevitably entailed surveillance that brought clinicians into new relationships with those for whom they cared. Among the most extensively discussed concerns about the widespread use of antiretrovirals in South Africa centered on the question of whether poor, sometimes illiterate patients would be able to sustain the level of adherence necessary for such medications to be effective; to prevent the development of resistant viral strains that would be far more difficult and far more expensive to treat.

At his Western Cape clinics, which by mid-2006 were providing ART to 11,000 people, Ashraf Grimwood introduced a cadre of patient advocates, nonclinicians who at once supported and monitored their clients.

> One patient advocate looks after 20 patients for their intensive phase of therapy, the first six months. They do home visits. Once a person goes onto therapy, they do intensive monitoring for the first week. They go

and visit every day. Once they're happy that there are no side effects, they then go every week for the first two months and then after that every fortnight and then once a month. If they're happy that things are fine after six months, then it's once-a-month telephone calls, or the odd visit. But they know the people they will look after. They're telling us how many people are living in the house, who have they disclosed to, what is the issue around disclosure, how many kids are on support grants, how many are not, what's the issue around food insecurity, housing security, domestic violence, drug abuse, and alcohol.

In the township of Guguletu, Linda-Gail Bekker used her "army of counselors," who were drawn from the pool of patients under care.

We have what we call a "doctor-lite" system—a little medical doctor input and much more of the layperson's input. Every patient is assigned a counselor. The counselors do all the treatment readiness training, so doctors and nurses are completely uninvolved in that. The patients very soon get to know these faces and have recognized that they are extremely knowledgeable people who know as much as anyone else about the antiretrovirals, and have come to trust them. They do the home visit; they get to know the family and get questions answered at home. They send messages back to the database. And it helps us keep tabs on our pill counts. There's an empathy, because the counselors are living with the virus; they themselves are taking tablets. And so I think it's been very effective.

But, however important counselors and other clinical staff were, those who began to create ART programs realized that ultimately they had to depend on the patients and their intimate networks for long-term compliance. That meant, at a minimum, that patients had to accept the clinicians' understanding of HIV infection and its treatment. As he prepared for the rollout to reach his rural hospital, Bernhard Gaede thought about the problems he had encountered with adherence to TB medication, which, unlike HIV, required no more than a year of treatment.

There are a lot of traditional beliefs around how the body works and also around HIV. One of the biggest indicators of whether a person is going to be compliant with a six-month course of treatment is whether they believe they have TB or not. Is it a traditional diagnosis, where somebody has been poisoned? Then, if one just says, "Take these medicines," as soon as they feel better, they leave the tablets. If somebody doesn't believe that they have HIV, it's very difficult to say, "OK, take this medicine, and you'll be fine." If you don't believe it is HIV, or if you don't believe that HIV works the way that it works, you are going to be noncompliant. That's the way it is.

Even patients who accepted the causal role of HIV often lacked the ability to understand adequately why strict adherence was so critical, why they had to take drugs once they no longer felt sick. Caroline Armstrong, who during training in Edinburgh, Scotland, knew that she wanted to work in Africa, now had to confront the implications of a deep cultural divide.

> When you don't come from a background with a little bit of science
> at school or generally a culture where it's understood, it's very difficult to
> explain terms. Resistance is particularly difficult to explain. Nobody un-
> derstands why missing a dose or two is really a problem. We have to think of
> ways to put it into culture-specific language, and I don't think we've
> done that yet.

Paradoxically, then, success in getting patients to take their medications as prescribed required more than following doctors' orders. The hierarchical relationship itself between doctors and poor patients in South Africa could represent an impediment, according to Linda-Gail Bekker.

> Patients often are unsophisticated; they don't have opportunities to be
> on Web sites and read things. And we have, in the past, had a very pa-
> ternalistic approach. "I know what's best for you and you do what I say, but
> if you don't understand it, it's your problem." But I think HIV has
> turned that on its head, because we're saying to people, "It's your re-
> sponsibility. You have this illness where you need to take the drug for life.
> We need you to own your disease." I'm not sure it's happening every-
> where, but certainly in our clinics, we are saying we have to empower these
> folk to, first of all, understand what's wrong with them, realize their re-
> sponsibility, come on as equal partners. And that can only happen through
> a process of education.

Nevertheless, expert clinical judgment remained central to assuring strict compliance with drug regimens. Concern that excessive alcohol and drug use might affect adherence led most clinics to screen carefully for such behaviors. In some settings, evidence of alcohol or drug problems could lead to a delay in treatment. In more extreme circumstances, treatment might be interrupted. In the Northern Cape, Eula Mothibi felt she had to act decisively, given the high prevalence of alcoholism she encountered there.

> This province is very poor, very sparse. The only form of leisure is alco-
> hol, so there's a very high alcoholism rate in the province; this province has
> the highest national figures for fetal alcohol syndrome. So that is one of the
> criteria for antiretroviral therapy, that people should cut down their
> drinking. I actually say, "You must stop. Please, try to stop before we begin

the drugs." It's not really just punitive. I'm not just saying, "Go home! You'll never get the drugs," but "You know you've got an option. Come back when you feel you are ready to take it." And then marijuana— there's a lot of cannabis smoking in the region that goes on, and other illicit drugs are coming through, so we encourage people that they must try and stop. We will exclude from treatment, but we keep on seeing them, and we offer ongoing counseling. The counselors will say, "Your CD4s are low, you're going to get sick very soon. It's in your hands. If you want the treatment, it's up to you. You have to stop." And most people do stop. They do stop. But I don't know for how long. Most do stop one or two months, but once they get better, I'm just worried that they will go back and drink.

At McCord Hospital, Henry Sunpath noted, "We try to be as nonjudgmental as possible. But if we see there are confounding factors like substance abuse or psychiatric problems, then in some instances we may advise stopping altogether."

Some clinicians adopted a wait-and-see attitude. Working at a clinic in Vulindlela, a small, rural community miles from her office at the Nelson R. Mandela School of Medicine in Durban, Kogie Naidoo believed that denying treatment to those who were dependent on alcohol was unethical. At the same time, she acknowledged that the evidence made it clear that such individuals were "poor pill takers."

You always can do teaching and counseling. Our policy is that, if a patient is nonadherent once they've been put onto the program, we give him a chance; but if he's showing a pattern of nonadherence, and in our judgment we're doing him more harm than good, then we stop ART altogether. That's the best you can do for him.

Acknowledging that alcohol use could well pose a barrier to successful ART that might be beyond the individual's ability to change, Linda-Gail Bekker faced questions about what she, as a clinician, had an obligation to do.

What do you do with the known alcoholic? How do you patch those people up so that they will actually manage their treatment sufficiently? In a way, we remain a little bit paternalistic. We can't adopt the attitude, "Well, it's your life," or "I'm going to give you these pills and if you choose to take them badly, it's your problem." There isn't a single Alcoholics Anonymous [group] in the whole district. So should I say to somebody, "Before I start you on treatment, I really want you to assure me that you've given up on alcohol," yet I provide no resources for him on how? Our antiretroviral clinics have to provide that kind of support as well.

Faced with a need to buffer and support their patients, many also believed it crucial to pierce the secrecy that so often surrounded AIDS. As an expression of paternalistic regard, many clinics routinely insisted that patients disclose news of their infection to at least one other person, someone who might support them physically and psychologically. Bernhard Gaede referred to a slogan he used to motivate his rural patients. " 'Out of the panty drawer, out on the kitchen table!' That's where the antiretrovirals need to be, so that everybody knows and people can remind you."

Some clinics made disclosure mandatory, compelling patients to choose between openly avowing they had a stigmatized condition or forgoing ART. Bekker, so flexible in other respects, was uncompromising about the need for individuals to reveal their disease in order to boost their chances of taking the drugs on schedule.

> We have been fairly forceful in saying to people, "You need to have disclosed to at least one other person. Secrecy, to the point that you are the only individual who knows about this, means that it's going to become inordinately difficult for you to take the tablets." It's different if you live in a penthouse apartment on Park Avenue in New York, but few people in our communities have that kind of luxury. They're usually living in a one- or two-bedroom house that's little more than a shack, and there are five to ten other people living with them. The scenario of secretly taking tablets for the rest of your life in that situation means that usually you don't do very well, in our experience.
>
> All the counselors have disclosed, many of them quite openly. Patients recognize that their lives didn't crash and burn because they did that, and the counselors also come and say, "If you need help to do that, we'll sit with you."

In Kimberley, Eula Mothibi, a self-described "bulldozer," was equally emphatic about disclosure.

> Some people might feel it's not right to force people to disclose, but I strongly feel that this is an important issue for a husband or wife. You must tell them before I feel OK about giving you treatment. If I disclose to my parents, family, brother, then I get their support. And I haven't, not even once, come across somebody who said, "I told my mother—or brother or family member—and they shunned me." When people disclose, they get the support.

In Durban, Raziya Bobat reported that the pediatric clinic at King Edward VIII also made it mandatory for mothers to disclose their own status.

> The mum must disclose to a second caregiver or adult, so that if she gets sick, somebody else takes over the treatment of the child. We've even

had mums who bring in fellow churchgoers; the church provides that support group for the mothers.

But not all clinics required disclosure. For some, it was a moral question: the unfairness of holding access to life-saving medication as ransom. For others, such coercion was simply counterproductive. The willingness to forgo compulsory disclosure was in some important measure informed by the fact that the rollout itself seemed to make self-revelation more common. In rural KwaZulu-Natal, in a setting that had been characterized by pervasive secrecy some years earlier, Bernhard Gaede discovered that many had become more forthcoming about their HIV status. He and his colleagues found that when they raised the issue of disclosure,

> we get this completely incredulous look, as if to say, "But everybody at home knows; how do you mean?" Quite a few people come with their partners, and because you come in one by one, I ask them, and they say, "Yes, my wife is next." The majority of people that come for CD4 counts at the moment have disclosed to at least one person at home. Probably half of them have disclosed to the whole family or to more than one person at home. So there is much greater openness now than there had been before.

In the first flush of the rollout, doctors noted high levels of compliance. Bekker reported that 95 percent of her patients in Guguletu were taking their doses of medication. Ashraf Grimwood found that 93 percent of his patients in a network of Western Cape clinics had undetectable viral loads, and seven of every ten tested had rising CD4 counts. In Durban, 80 percent of McCord patients were adherent, according to Henry Sunpath, while in nearby Vulindlela, in the KwaZulu-Natal midlands, May Mkhize reported that her rate was 90 percent or better.

Even as their initial experiences with adherence were strikingly successful, clinicians fretted about the future. ART treatment was lifelong. Wouldn't patients suffer from complacency, or what one doctor called "treatment fatigue," once they were symptom-free and feeling healthy? For May Mkhize, who had been practicing medicine since 1982, the experience of treating tuberculosis, which required only 6–12 months of drug therapy, gave her pause. "Generally, we've had poor adherence to TB treatment, and that's my nightmare about ART. We've given people some form of information and training, but I'm not sure how good that's going to be."

And how effective would clinic adherence programs be as the number of patients grew? At Grey's Hospital, Caroline Armstrong observed, "Since we've been putting large numbers of people on every day, we've lost a little bit in terms of excellence of compliance." In addition, how committed to patient compliance would the newly approved ART clinics prove to be in the absence of historically dedicated teams of clinicians? Speaking about Jerry Coovadia, an esteemed senior colleague, Linda-Gail Bekker confessed:

It's hard work. Jerry always reminds me, "You know, you're champions at this." I think he's right. All the people running the clinic are passionate, and they're devoted to making sure people take their pills, and we spend hours thinking about strategies to try and enhance this. The challenge for us is, how do we roll out that kind of enthusiasm across the whole country, across the continent?

Resurrections, Reconstitutions, Reactions, and Recoveries: Patients' Responses to ART

As they watched young women and men return to productive lives, Lazarus-like recoveries could be enormously moving and satisfying for veterans of the AIDS epidemic. In Kimberley, Eula Mothibi recalled one such patient.

> She was weighing 24 kilograms. She's a young mother. She's 32. She's got a small child of about 3 or 4 years. She couldn't walk. Her mother was looking after her. And she'd been a very productive woman. She was a health aid instructor. It just happens sometimes, some patients, your heart just goes out for them, and for some reason you pray for them. I don't pray! But sometimes I just say, "God, just let her live for the next two weeks. Let her start the drug." And she did. And she came to me and said, "I have to go back to work! Sign my papers!" It's just incredible. That kind of thing makes one feel good. And I think as well, The patients, they don't say it to me, but it must be a miracle, almost. And quite a lot of them come in like that, the females especially. "Doctor, I'm well now. I'm going to be well forever!" And I know in my own heart that they're going to stick to the drugs, barring side effects. They will take the drugs, because they've looked death in the eye.

Not all recoveries went smoothly and swiftly, however. Patients were susceptible to a reconstitution syndrome in which dormant pathogens were, paradoxically, stimulated by a more vibrant immune system. Paul Kocheleff described such a patient at his Grey's Hospital clinic, a foreman on a farm who began antiretroviral treatment when his CD4 count stood at 2.

> After a period of antiretroviral drugs, saying, "I'm fine, it's good, no side effects, I can work," he started complaining of tiredness, pain in the gastric area, sometimes vomiting, and his weight was going down, going down. An investigation showed that he had a disseminated tuberculosis that he didn't have before starting antiretroviral drugs. That was probably immune reconstitution syndrome, associated with a huge psychological

disturbance because his wife died, despite the medication. For a few weeks, in October, November, his weight was going down. I didn't know how it would go. He was very concerned and trying to take his medication stoically. And on the last visit that he had a few days ago, his weight is going up and he's smiling. Very probably, in a short time, he will be able to start working.

Tony Moll had seen on a small scale what ART could do because of his ongoing Yale University research project. He was, nevertheless, profoundly affected when the totality of the impact of the rollout on his poor patients became clear. Normally emotionally unruffled, Moll, who speaks in careful, measured tones, wept as he recalled the scene.

Just before Christmas 2004, the staff organized, without me knowing, a kind of little party, and they invited patients that had been a couple of months on antiretroviral therapy, and they had prepared little presents for them as well. And I was just carrying on with my normal routine, and they said, "Hey, Doctor, come and join us for something." And I came, and there were patients sitting there—not many, maybe 15 or so—and our nursing staff, and they gave me an envelope. "What's inside this envelope?" They said, "Those are the latest CD4 counts and viral loads of the patients here." And jeepers, the party started, people were singing and dancing. And then they got me to read out the CD4 counts and viral loads. It was incredible, because they'd come up from 10 or 15. The viral loads were undetectable. And there were people there that should have died. The experience of seeing young mothers who really would have been dead if it wasn't for antiretrovirals, seeing them being able to look after their children again and just look so good. Their skin was good, and they were healthy and energetic and full of life. If you saw them in the village, you would never think, wow, that's a dying AIDS patient.

In Cape Town, Paul Roux reported that at an orphanage to which he sent HIV-infected children none had died over the last year. "The favorite game at Nazareth House used to be 'let's play funeral.' It bothered me, but the psychologists seemed to think it was a healthy thing. They're not doing that any more, because funerals aren't happening."

But for many, access to drugs came too late. At Cape Town's Tygerberg Hospital, Mark Cotton spoke of losing the race to save such patients.

The preparatory process can take a few weeks to get them treated, and we've seen kids deteriorate in front of our eyes. We're learning that sometimes you have to rush into it and just treat and worry about the consequences afterwards, because we've seen some kids just go down very quickly. It was incredibly frustrating to lose kids when there was no treatment; it's equally hard now.

But We're Still Hungry

In the years when President Mbeki and his health minister had publicly railed against ART, they repeatedly asserted that it was poverty and not a virus that most determined the patterns of disease suffered by South Africa's Black majority. Now that the scaling up of antiretroviral therapy had begun in the public sector, advocates had to confront the ways that material deprivation did, in fact, affect treatment. Simply getting to a clinic could be very difficult, as May Mkhize, herself a product of impoverished, rural Mpumalanga Province, emphasized.

> Remember, the clinics are far away from them. The patients have to attend the clinic to be tested, and then they must attend the adherence support program. People don't have the money for food; they don't have money for transport. But they have to, because if you don't attend adherence support, you will not be enrolled for therapy.

At Mosvold Hospital, which by mid-2006 would have 250 patients on ART, Ann Barnard saw how profound poverty could undercut antiretroviral therapy.

> One of the biggest needs that we are seeing with the home-based care patients is that they don't have any food, and to give antiretrovirals without food [can have awful consequences]. We then compared that idea with TB medicine, where we find that they are vomiting their pills as it is.

Ironically, as their immune systems rebounded, many patients on ART found their appetites becoming rapacious, straining their already slender stocks of food. In rural Vulindlela, Kogie Naidoo reported:

> In the early days of treatment, we see patients weekly, and you're seeing this person starting to gain weight in leaps and bounds. So there's a sense of euphoria. They come in complaining because their families don't want them any more; they're eating the entire household budget away. It's a real issue! There's no food left for the children or the old people. The vegetable gardens alongside their homes are not enough to sustain their appetite, and they come to you now with other problems. "Please help me with food. I want your tablets, but I'm hungry."

Effective treatment could exacerbate the burdens of poverty in other ways as well. Caroline Armstrong discovered that the very success of treatment was undercutting the eligibility of her patients in Pietermaritzburg for the social service supports they still required.[11]

> Most of these people have been on disability pensions. But if they're blossoming on antiretrovirals, they need to come off their disability pensions. They say to us, "But why not? I've still got HIV." That's very difficult for us because we want them to get the money, we want them to be able to eat and to live comfortably. We don't provide food. There is the protein antimalnutrition scheme, which provides milk and beans to really underweight people. But then of course, once they're on their antiretrovirals, their weight picks up.

The Decline of Stigma?

Advocates for treatment and many health care providers had hoped, even predicted, that the transformative power of ART, its ability to forestall or prevent the degenerative and fatal consequences of HIV, would lift the heavy burden of stigma surrounding the disease. As they observed their patients, many believed that their assumptions had proved to be largely correct, at least in the initial period of scaling up access to treatment. The increasing willingness of patients to reveal their infection to others within their intimate circles testified to the success of antiretroviral drugs, both medically and socially. From her observations at McCord Hospital, Helga Holst saw a slow weakening of HIV-related stigma with the introduction of ART.

> I think stigma is diminishing as patients are put onto treatment and as they are getting better. Amongst our HIV-infected staff, they may not openly say that they are positive, but people will comment, "Oh, you've gained weight and you're looking so much better." Amongst our patients, employers are much more willing to help their domestic workers that are HIV positive and say, "We'll see them through this illness. We'll help them with their ART. We'll be their supervisors. They're going to keep their jobs."

And in Vulindlela, May Mkhize believed that stigma had lost some of its impact.

> You know, there's still a lot of stigma surrounding this disease. People are even afraid of coming to the center because that site is associated with HIV. But once a patient plucks up the courage and comes, and you check them and you start them on ART, and they feel the difference it makes, not only in themselves but they're looking at other patients who were very sick and who kept on coming to our site, and they can see that the patients are better; it makes a lot of difference. It even makes other people decide, "I'm not afraid to say I've got the infection."

But stigma had not vanished. At King Edward VIII Hospital, Kogie Naidoo noted that, even though her clinic patients were seeking out testing and antiretroviral treatment, many continued to fear the consequences of revealing their status. "Stigma still exists. Disclosure is still a problem among relationships. I'm still having a hard time convincing people to speak to somebody about their status, to get support from their families and friends and among their peers." Even within the same clinic, some felt free to be open while others continued to seek the protection of secrecy. At Baragwanath Hospital, Tammy Meyers observed:

> I'm sitting in a clinic where all the people have been tested already. I'll be
> sitting with patients who are happy for their children to be talking
> about HIV freely in front of other people. So I think that has improved. Yet
> there are many people who still haven't disclosed to anybody else in the
> family. There still is a lot of stigma. My sense is that it's less than it used to
> be; there's a much more positive attitude. There's still a long way to go.

In the context of the lingering hesitancy and their patients' fears, and of the potency of the stigma that still attached to HIV, the decision of Nelson Mandela to announce in January 2005 that his eldest son had died of an AIDS-related disease took on much meaning. At a press conference, the former president challenged his nation by saying, "Let us give publicity to HIV/AIDS and not hide it, because the only way of making it appear to be a normal disease just like TB, like cancer, is always to come out and say somebody has died of AIDS."[12] Although moved by Mandela's candor, Linda-Gail Bekker wished, for the sake of public instruction, that he had made an even fuller revelation.

> He will never know how important it was for him—and I'm sure it was very
> painful and more painful for his family—to have come forward and dis-
> closed what happened to his son, Makgatho. It was very important, be-
> cause suddenly this is not so terrible. It would even have been better if he'd
> said his son had taken treatment for so many years, and here are the reasons
> why the treatment failed. I think people still wonder why he didn't get
> antiretrovirals or what went wrong. But those are the kinds of stories we
> need, so that the communities actually feel OK that somebody's attending
> an antiretroviral clinic.

Shifting Professional Perceptions?

Were claims about the diminution of stigma matched by observations of the shifting attitudes and actions of those who managed public health care institutions? Paul Nijs, head of the communicable disease clinic at Edendale Hospital, reported in early 2005 that, since the beginning of the rollout, he had never seen a hospital superintendent or manager at the clinic. At Baragwanath, Alan Karstaedt, who oversaw the vast adult clinic, found the hospital administration as unresponsive as ever. "We're supposed to have management meetings, but there have been only two since the beginning of the rollout." Tammy Meyers, his colleague, found the administration's lack of interest to be a continuing impediment to her efforts. "After the rollout," she said:

> We never had any communication with the hospital administration
> about what they were going to do—were they were going to employ extra
> people? We were running out of space, and I kept desperately trying to
> say, "Let's try and set up meetings with the administration," and nothing
> ever happened.

The story was not universally bleak, however. In some hospitals, administrators became markedly more responsive. At Cape Town's Tygerberg Hospital, which Mark Cotton had earlier characterized as steeped in Afrikaner hierarchy and rigidity and generally antipathetic toward his HIV interventions, the provincial government's strong support of ART transformed management's stance. "In this hospital, as soon as something becomes official—in other words, once they receive a directive from head office to, say, start treating with antiretrovirals—they do it. Then it's no longer an issue."

And at Grey's Hospital, where Paul Kocheleff had documented years of administrative indifference toward the AIDS service, he began to receive new managerial attention.

> The interest has increased a lot with the rollout of antiretroviral drugs.
> I don't know if it's because the administration was as excited as we were to
> start antiretroviral drugs or if it was some political effect, but that's not
> important. What's important is the interest of the management has im-
> proved really a lot. They cannot always solve the problems, but they
> know the problems, and we can discuss them. And that never happened
> before. Never!

At the same time, the posture of clinical nihilism that had so informed attitudes toward patients with HIV began to shift. Indicative of the changing climate was the attitude of those responsible for intensive care units who, in the past, almost uniformly considered HIV patients to be ineligible for admission. At King Edward VIII, the advent of antiretroviral therapy had, according to Raziya Bobat, opened the ICU to the children she treated.

> Previously, we would have said, "This kid needs ventilation, but he's HIV
> positive." The response would be "There's not much we're going to be able
> to do. We'd rather keep the bed for somebody else." It doesn't happen

now. There was a kid, and the question came up, "Should we ventilate?" and the answer was yes, because we can now offer him antiretroviral therapy.

Umesh Lalloo, a pulmonologist who directed the adult ICU at King Edward VIII, was more skeptical than Bobat, his wife, and noted a lingering antipathy toward the treatment of critically sick people with HIV.

I think many people would be somewhat less reluctant to take on HIV-infected patients, knowing that there's an opportunity for access to antiretroviral treatment. I think that's beginning to change. I'm not sure how dramatically. Some of my colleagues are still unwilling. I had a patient two days ago who was refused admission to another ICU because he had Guillain-Barré syndrome with HIV. We readily took on the patient because our experience, irrespective of antiretroviral availability, is HIV-infected patients with that syndrome have an excellent outcome in the ICU.

Lalloo's response to his colleagues' misapprehensions was strong and deeply felt, in part because of their arrogance and clinical ignorance. "I get very angry. I think doctors have got to be extremely careful that we don't play God." But his anger revealed a raw nerve, connecting the current rejection of HIV patients with the experiences he had under apartheid.

We mustn't kid ourselves: there is still in the country a lot of racial bias around. I'm not sure how individuals think, but I wouldn't be surprised if people make their decision, not only on HIV, but on race as well. I grew up practicing intensive care medicine in a very racist environment, where a Black patient would be denied intensive care, but the white patient would get free access to it. And I've had personal experience with it. My mother had severe asthma, had a cardiac arrest, and needed ventilation, and my ICU was full. And there was another ICU in a white hospital that had beds, and intensivists, despite knowing me, refused to accept her. I had to use a broken ventilator to ventilate my mother myself, yet there were two beds available in that ICU. I think things have changed, but that doesn't mean that it doesn't occur at all. That still exists.

Eula Mothibi also drew upon her experiences of recurrent racism. At Kimberley Hospital, the head of the ICU still rejected HIV-infected patients. But Mothibi forced him to admit her charges.

If I want my patients in the ICU, then I get my patients in there. The junior doctors know, if there's an HIV patient who's very sick and they think the person needs the ICU, they will just call me so I can bulldoze my way into the ICU. I think that is the only way to do it. And then I will also try to educate the ICU staff. I say, "This person has got pneumonia. It's not the HIV that's going to kill him, and you know that pneumonia is a treatable condition. And apart from that, I've got antiretrovirals."

Mothibi ascribed her toughness to her own experiences growing up in a white- and male-dominated South Africa. "It goes back to our history. I'm a Black woman, and I'm a Black physician. There are very few Black physicians in the country. I care for the patients, and I wouldn't just go there playing around."

Changes occurred as well in contexts less extreme than those involving ICUs. Paul Kocheleff observed a shift among his clinical colleagues.

Very few doctors were interested in working in the clinic before the rollout. They were interested to come for a few weeks, but not really to work over the long run. Now that we have antiretroviral drugs, they are really interested, interested to come and to learn, and not laughing about the idea of working for a long time in the clinic.

At Baragwanath, Tammy Meyers had also begun to see long-hoped-for changes.

People are starting to think differently. Even in the wards, the doctors who work with us try to keep up a big presence to show that the patients are treated like they should be; and I think that helps, seeing that there are people who go out and put as much effort as they can into these children. More and more, I'm coming across people who are actually coming to see me and, you know, "What can we do here? How can I help with this patient?"

But, as in the case with ICU care, the story was not uniformly positive, and resistance to caring for patients with HIV lingered. Raziya Bobat was uncharacteristically critical about the surgeons at her hospital. While more doctors had begun to ask:

"What can we do for patients?" the surgeons—that's a different kettle of fish altogether. Oh, we've had a lot of difficulty. We couldn't even get biopsies on kids who were HIV positive. I'm not sure whether they've changed their attitude.

Like Bobat, Paul Roux, who cared for children with AIDS, could remark that at Groote Schuur in Cape Town he still had difficulty getting children into the cancer service, and that, as a consequence, "We've got kids with Kaposi's sarcoma who would otherwise be receiving chemotherapy in the oncology unit, but we give the chemotherapy in my unit."

"A Drop in the Ocean?" The Impact of ART on the Epidemic

In January 2005, less than a year after the start of the government's rollout, clinicians looked back on their initial efforts. Raziya Bobat pointed to signs of a decline in HIV-infected babies on the wards after several years of prescribing the drug nevirapine for mothers in labor.

> We see the impact in our wards. Whereas previously we'd have kids almost every day where we were seeing PCP, we don't see that any more. And we're seeing fewer kids coming in the first few months [of life] than we did before, and that's definitely the impact of the mother-to-child transmission prevention program.

But Bobat's experience was exceptional, a function of the ways in which nevirapine reduced the risk of HIV infection in newborns. The rollout had not yet produced similar decreases in the burden on the adult medical wards of hospitals. According to Paul Kocheleff:

> I couldn't say that we have had a change. We are very proud to have 700 people on treatment, but what is that if we know that there are—nobody knows exactly—probably a million or two who should be on treatment? It's evident that the 700 people on treatment are only a small part of the epidemic. And all the other people who are HIV positive, severely immunocompromised, are such a big number. It will take a long time before we see people who don't need any more to be admitted. It's not like in Europe or the United States, where the number of patients was so limited that, after a short time, you could see that there's an impact. Here, we have a small number identified, and we have a huge number not identified. One day they will become ill, and if they have complications, they will be admitted here in Grey's Hospital.

The numbers reached by the rollout more than 15 months after it had been announced were, said Ashraf Grimwood, who had been involved in planning the rollout, but a bare fraction of those dying. "It's the 700, 800, 900 people dying per day. It's the 380,000 people expected to die in a year, and the 5.6 million people that are positive, and the 560,000 that need to be on therapy as we speak." For Bongani Thembela, the effect remained "a drop in the ocean."

And so there was no let-up in the dying and suffering that had come to define AIDS. For Henry Sunpath, it was a situation that was likely to prevail for years at McCord and other hospitals.

> When I walk into my ward and 60–70 percent of the patients are so ill, it's like being in an intensive care unit. So the whole nature of HIV care

hasn't changed that dramatically. I think it's still early. We still face those issues of people dying, having to deal with it all the time. That really does continue to take a toll on us emotionally, psychologically. Maybe ten years down the line, we would not be having much need for hospice care. The epidemic is out there in very advanced stages, and even if ART reaches a significant number of people, there are going to be millions of people who are still going to need terminal care. You know, by 2015, we expect up to 8 million people to die. That's a fact.

Looking Back: The Wages of Engagement

The commencement of ART so late in the epidemic, when so many patients had died and when the escalation in the number of cases continued unabated, was a bittersweet moment for many AIDS doctors. The years of struggle against the disease, colleagues, administrators, and the national government had had a profound personal effect on these men and women. A few had become particularly well known, because they had undertaken important clinical trials or, sometimes at personal risk, had publicly voiced their outrage at the South African government's approach to AIDS under President Mbeki. But most of these clinicians, even those who had participated in the anti-apartheid movement, had confronted the AIDS epidemic mainly as professionals in offices, clinics, and hospitals, ministering to the patients who came to them. And it was mainly from within the crucible of AIDS treatment that they viewed the effect of the epidemic on themselves. Called to their task just as the struggle against apartheid was ending, many found that the epidemic had enriched and deepened their lives as doctors. For Paul Nijs, who was willing to treat patients whom others tried to avoid, the AIDS epidemic "offered me an opportunity to be the doctor that I thought I could be."

Like Nijs, Eric Goemaere was a Belgian expatriate. He had spent his career abroad, organizing the medical responses of Médecins sans Frontières to large-scale catastrophes and displaced populations. Now, in middle age, he found AIDS personally and professionally transformative, reintroducing him to direct patient care.

I never doubted I have got the rightness of what we are doing here. The most important change is this commitment, this personal commitment that this implies. You are confronted with an individual and you restart individual relationships. It's probably one of the best things that happened to me in my professional life.

Having come to AIDS before many others because he was a gay man caring for gay men with AIDS in the 1980s, Steven Miller struggled to find words that could capture the impact of HIV on his understanding of what it meant to be a doctor. He wanted to avoid the religious tones that came so easily to many in South Africa, but he could not avoid speaking of "meaning." "HIV highlighted for me a new definition of healing. It taught me how important it was to create good in someone's life." And so, despite the fact that he had been among the first in the country to prescribe ART in his relatively privileged practice, he found, "There's nothing in scientific medicine that creates for me the same feeling of satisfaction or fulfillment" as that intangible goal.

Even for those who had not experienced the epidemic as transformative, the encounter with AIDS was commonly seen as deepening their understanding of the worlds within which they worked. Paul Roux, now in his mid-50s, who had pioneered pediatric HIV care at Groote Schuur Hospital unassisted by its academically oriented professional staff, found that the AIDS epidemic had served to confirm his sense of what it was to be a doctor. "I don't think the experience of this epidemic has changed me. I still see myself as a comforter of the sick. What's happened is that events seem to have affirmed my assessment of myself." But Roux, an Afrikaner working in what was, under apartheid, one of the premier white public hospitals, found his social world view broadened by the epidemic.

> I think way back, before access to antiretrovirals, a big penny that
> dropped was that I used to think of HIV people as being definite types, a
> different sort, a different set of humans; but the penny that dropped
> was that there's a parent looking after a sick child with HIV, and there's no
> difference between this person and other parents.

Working in her internationally funded treatment program in Guguletu had provided Linda-Gail Bekker with the opportunity to witness fortitude, which she in the end could draw upon as she faced the challenges of AIDS work.

> I have learned so much from young people who are coping with the
> most awesome tragedies in their lives and yet rise above it. They've looked
> death in its face and that's what one draws strength from. I have had
> that opportunity to see the strength that human beings can come up with
> under this very difficult situation. I have learned that being a medical
> doctor in this epidemic, in this situation, means that I have to draw on
> every resource, every talent and skill that I have at my disposal to fight the
> virus, to fight policy, to fight politics.

AIDS also propelled some doctors in directions they might not have otherwise pursued. Tony Moll stressed that the epidemic had bound him professionally and personally to the bare rural villages in which he had begun his career.

> I wouldn't have stayed at the Church of Scotland Hospital, actually, if it
> wasn't for the epidemic. It was the challenges of the epidemic and the
> reward of seeing that I can make a difference that has actually kept me here.

Otherwise, I suppose, I would have gone on to specialize or taken on some other challenges. I've been offered jobs in other places that would have—can I say—materially been a promotion. But it was more attractive to me just to stay here in the bush—my family is happy here—and to see a project go through and help more people that wouldn't otherwise have been able to benefit from help. Because this is very much a forgotten part of the geography over here. It's a rural, out-of-the-way place.

A long-standing member of the African National Congress, May Mkhize, who had spent years in exile with her husband in Swaziland and Zimbabwe, saw her AIDS work as another form of personal and political commitment. Nevertheless, had she not encountered the epidemic, doctoring would have been very different for her.

Maybe I would have found more joy. My joy is actually making people feel better, and that has not been the case in terms of the epidemic. There was a time when we lost hope. I know we are starting to gain hope because we've got the antiretrovirals. They will make a big difference in people's lives. But I must say that the epidemic did affect me as a person. It was very depressing actually; it was. But even within that depression, a person had to go on.

But not all doctors could frame their experiences in such terms. David Johnson, who, like Miller, had a private AIDS practice, was appalled by the inequities that characterized HIV care in South Africa. He was "angry that people get sick, and that they are not treated in time. Angry that people come in when it's too late. Angry that there aren't the resources that should be there. Angry that there are people who cannot afford the drugs." Deep frustration, spawned by the spotty progress of treatment in the public sector and gnawing feelings of clinical powerlessness, led Bongani Thembela to seek out medical opportunities that would no longer directly involve him in treating AIDS patients.

I think I've seen too many people die. Some of them have been people who are close to me, like relatives. It's reached a point where, if I see a patient who I know needs antiretrovirals and I realize that this patient is only going to be assessed in April or May next year, it's impossible for me to function. It just becomes impossible for me to function. I can no longer look at patients in the face and tell them, "You will get treatment but probably in May next year." I cannot do that any more. I don't want to do that any more, because I don't think it's justified.

In a nation whose social fabric would be profoundly affected by the HIV epidemic for years to come and where doctors and nurses would, willingly or not, be engulfed by the need to care for people with AIDS, those who came first to the challenge inevitably created narratives—both individual and collective—that explained why they chose to act as they had. Their accounts would at the same time explain why others had failed to see in AIDS so defining a moral and medical challenge. Speaking to her colleagues, Linda-Gail Bekker drew on such a narrative to both inspire and guide.

> My words to them were, "You're sitting in this room. You've self-selected yourselves. You're here because you believe that you should be here and you have the heart for HIV-infected people. You have to remember you've left behind the rest of the medical profession, and some of those people will be sympathetic but a good number of them feel nothing about this epidemic. That's the reality. You have to have an understanding of that. You've got to work on the premise that you are somewhat unusual. And then you've got to bring your colleagues up gently and use patience with them; you've got to lead by example."

In Medias Res

The year 2004 marked a milestone in the encounter with AIDS in South Africa. Ten years after the election of Nelson Mandela as president and after years of grim experiences, there was, at last, a ray of hope: patients might get treated, and for them there was the prospect of life where, before, HIV had meant a death sentence; more clinicians might become involved in providing treatment; and the burdens of stigma might give way to greater transparency and disclosure. In Cape Town, Bekker spoke enthusiastically about the moment.

> I think we're in the most amazing time in our lives now in this country. I can only describe it as a human experiment because I actually don't know where it's going to end up. But as this thing unfolds, it's incredibly inspiring and such a privilege to be part of it.

As he celebrated the enrollment of his 500th patient in mid-2006, Bernhard Gaede, who had felt so despairing two years earlier, before he had access to antiretroviral therapy, said:

> For me, this has been one of the most wonderful things to see. For many people starting antiretrovirals, it has been a journey of facing fear, denial, and uncertainty and finding new strength and direction in life. A significant number have made decisions about their relationships, about what they want to do in life, about what their goals are, who they want to be. One woman quit her job as a waitress to complete her matric. When I asked her why, she said, "I don't want to be a waitress for the rest of my life."

But even as they still dared to hope, those who were most committed were uncertain about when the worst would be over. For Glenda Gray, whose world view early on had been shaped by revolutionary fervor, hope was expressed as a millenarian wish.

> I became a pediatrician because I wanted to save children's lives and impact on child mortality and survival. And that's what I want to see. It's not going to happen in five years. But when I retire, one day, I want to say, "When I started my career, HIV reversed mortality in children, and when I ended my career, we're back to where we should have been."

More cautiously, Brian Brink, who had worked so assiduously to assure that the Anglo American Corporation would provide treatment to its workers, remained unsure about when the epidemic that had threatened to shatter the dream of a post-apartheid South Africa would be brought to heel.

> I still maintain we have not seen the worst of this epidemic by a long, long way. It's still coming. But my vision is that we can deal with AIDS. We can get on top of this epidemic, and we can arrive at a situation where it is not the central issue of the day. I wish we could get there soon. But I fear that, in my lifetime, we're not going to get there. I just see the people dying every day.

. . .

In mid-2006, more than a year after our last visit to South Africa, there were new reasons to despair and hope. At the biennial international AIDS conference, held in Toronto and attended by more than 30,000 delegates, the official South African booth displayed a basket of herbal remedies that the minister of health had put forth as an alternative to antiretroviral therapies; strikingly absent from the booth were any of the AIDS medicines the public sector had already begun to provide. Steven Lewis, the United Nations' special envoy on AIDS, was moved to publicly denounce South Africa, describing its policies as "worthy of a lunatic fringe."

Two months later, there were clear signs that the government of President Mbeki was ready to shed the policies that had been a source of derision in Toronto. Responsibility for managing the nation's AIDS program appears to have been transferred from the minister of health, there was a new willingness to work with groups such as the Treatment Action Campaign, and there were suggestions that the government would speed the rollout of ART. Leaders of TAC spoke of their "growing enthusiasm," in light of these changes. But with so many false starts and against a backdrop of shattered dreams, others were only ready to say, "Time will tell."

NOTES

Introduction

1. Leonard Thompson, *A History of South Africa*, rev. ed. (New Haven, Conn., and London: Yale University Press, 1995), 204–279.

2. Anthony Sampson, *Mandela: The Authorized Biography* (New York: Knopf, 1999).

3. Zena Stein and Anthony Zwi (eds.), "Action on AIDS in Southern Africa: Maputo Conference on Health in Transition in Southern Africa" (1990), unpublished report, 137.

4. Ibid., 136.

5. Hein Marais, *To the Edge: AIDS Review 2000* (Pretoria: Centre for the Study of AIDS, University of Pretoria, 2000), 4.

6. NACOSA, "A National AIDS Plan for South Africa, 1994–1995" (1994), unpublished report, 1.

7. "South African HIV/AIDS Statistics," http://www.avert.org/safricastats.htm (accessed 19 May 2006).

8. R. E. Dorrington, D. Bradshaw, L. Johnson, and D. Budlender, *The Demographic Impact of HIV/AIDS in South Africa: National Indicators for 2004* (Cape Town: Centre for Actuarial Research, South African Medical Research Council and Actuarial Society of South Africa, 2004), 8.

9. Ibid., 9.

10. Barbara A. Anderson and Heston E. Phillips, *Adult Mortality (Age 15–64) Based on Death Notification Data in South Africa: 1997–2004*, Report No. 03-09-05 (Pretoria: Statistics South Africa, 2006), xv.

11. Rob Dorrington, personal communication, February 26, 2007.

12. Samantha Power, "The AIDS Rebel," *New Yorker* 79 (2003): 54–67.

13. Nicoli Nattrass, "AIDS, Science and Governance: The Battle over Antiretroviral Therapy in Post-Apartheid South Africa" (19 March 2006), unpublished paper; Virginia van der Vliet, "South Africa Divided against AIDS: A Crisis of Leadership," in Kyle D. Kauffman and David L. Lindauer (eds.), *AIDS and South Africa: The Social Expression of a Pandemic* (New York: Palgrave Macmillan, 2004), 48–96.

14. Ronald Bayer and Gerald Oppenheimer, *AIDS Doctors: Voices from the Epidemic* (New York: Oxford University Press, 2000).

15. Shula Marks, *Divided Sisterhood: Race, Class and Gender in the South African Nursing Profession* (New York: St. Martin's, 1994), 138–213.

16. H. C. J. van Rensburg and S. R. Benatar, "The Legacy of Apartheid in Health and Health Care," *South African Journal of Sociology* 24 (1993): 105–106.

17. Solomon R. Benatar, "Medicine and Health Care in South Africa—Five Years Later," *New England Journal of Medicine* 325 (1991): 30.

18. Thompson, *A History of South Africa*, 187–240.

19. Allister Sparks, *The Mind of South Africa: The Story of the Rise and Fall of Apartheid* (Johannesburg and Cape Town: Ball, 1990).

20. H. C. J. van Rensburg (ed.), *Health and Health Care in South Africa* (Pretoria: Van Schaik, 2004), 81.

21. Karen Jochelson, *The Colour of Disease: Syphilis and Racism in South Africa, 1880–1950* (Oxford: Palgrave, 2001).

22. Shula Marks, "An Epidemic Waiting to Happen? The Spread of HIV/AIDS in South Africa: A Social and Historical Perspective," *African Studies* 61 (2002): 20.

23. Sidney L. Kark, "The Social Pathology of Syphilis in Africans," *South African Medical Journal* 23 (1949): 77–84.

24. Thompson, *A History of South Africa*, 203.

25. Randall Packard, *White Plague, Black Labor: Tuberculosis and the Political Economy of Health and Disease in South Africa* (Berkeley: University of California Press, 1989), 11; Marks, "An Epidemic Waiting to Happen?" 18.

26. Packard, *White Plague, Black Labor*, 287–291.

27. van Rensburg and Benatar, "The Legacy of Apartheid in Health and Health Care," 106.

28. Thompson, *A History of South Africa*, 279; van Rensburg and Benatar, "The Legacy of Apartheid in Health and Health Care," 106.

29. van Rensburg, *Health and Health Care in South Africa*, 80–83, 103.

30. Ibid., 83.

31. Given the length of the hospital's name, we will, like many current clinicians, refer to it in this book simply as Baragwanath Hospital.

32. van Rensburg and Benatar, "The Legacy of Apartheid in Health and Health Care," 102.

33. van Rensburg, *Health and Health Care in South Africa*, 83.

34. Marks, *Divided Sisterhood*, 198–199.

35. Ibid., 141.

36. Ibid., 136, 137, 172–178.

37. Aruna M. Kamath, "NAMDA 1982–1990: Mobilizing the Health Care Sector in the Fight against Apartheid" (June 2004), unpublished paper.

38. Ibid., 32.

39. van Rensburg, *Health and Health Care in South Africa*, 95.

40. Ibid.

41. Ibid.

42. Ibid., 94.

Chapter 1

1. Mark Gevisser, "A Different Fight for Freedom: A History of South African Lesbian and Gay Organizations from the 1950s to 1990s," in Mark Gevisser and Edwin Cameron (eds.), *Defiant Desire* (New York: Routledge, 1995), 14–88.

2. G. J. Ras, I. W. Simson, R. Anderson, O. W. Prozesky, and T. Hamersma, "Acquired Immunodeficiency Syndrome: A Report of 2 South African Cases," *South African Medical Journal* 64 (1983): 140–142.

3. F. H. N. Spracklen, R. G. Whittaker, W. B. Becker, M. L. B. Becker, C. M. Holmes, and P. C. Potter, "The Acquired Immune Deficiency Syndrome and Related Complex," *South African Medical Journal* 68 (1985): 143.

4. S. F. Lyons, B. D. Schoub, G. M. McGillivray, and R. Sher, "Sero-epidemiology of HTLV-III Antibody in Southern Africa," *South African Medical Journal* 67 (1985): 962.

5. Gevisser, "A Different Fight for Freedom," 35.

6. Ibid., 35.

7. Ibid., 70.

8. Ibid., 69–73.

9. S. L. Sellars, "Contraction of HIV Infection during Mutual Masturbation," *South African Medical Journal* 74 (1988): 187.

10. Belinda Beresford, "Clinic Head: Ban Gay People," *Mail and Guardian*, 22 June 2001, 2.

11. Gevisser, "A Different Fight for Freedom," 43.

12. "AIDS Panic Is Overstressed," *Link/Skakel* (February 1983): 1.

13. Ibid.

14. J. H. S. Gear, "Highlights of Medical Research at the South African Institute for Medical Research," *Adler Museum Bulletin* 16 (1990): 12–18.

15. R. Sher, "HIV Infection in South Africa, 1982–1988: A Review," *South African Medical Journal* 76 (1989): 314–318.

16. Edwin Cameron, *Witness to AIDS* (Cape Town: Tafelberg, 2005), 52.

17. "Gov't AIDS Chief Warns against Dangerous Hysteria," *Link/Skakel* (March 1985): 7.

18. "There Is No African AIDS, No Western AIDS, No Gay AIDS, No Heterosexual AIDS. There Is Only One AIDS," *Weekly Mail*, 5–12 May 1988, 15.

19. G. J. Knobel, Response, *South African Medical Journal* 80 (1991): 460.

20. B. N. Pitchford, "Guidelines on HIV Infection" (letter), *South African Medical Journal* 81 (1992): 171.

21. Bernard Rabinowitz, "The Great Hijack," *British Medical Journal* 313 (1996): 826.

22. "Survey Results: Sexual Behaviour Not Changed by AIDS Scare," *Exit* (August–September 1989): 3.

23. M. C. Botha, F. A. Neethling, I. Shai, et al., "Two Black South Africans with AIDS" (letter), *South African Medical Journal* 73 (1988): 132.

24. Sher, "HIV Infection in South Africa, 1982–1988," 314.

25. R. Sher, "Addendum," *South African Medical Journal* 76 (1989): 318.

26. R. A. Bobat, H. M. Coovadia, and I. M. Windsor, "Some Early Observations on HIV Infection in Children at King Edward VIII Hospital, Durban," *South African Medical Journal* 78 (1990): 524–527.

27. R. Schall, G. N. Padayachee, and D. Yach, "The Case for Surveillance in South Africa," *South African Medical Journal* 77 (1990): 324–325.

28. R. Schall and G. N. Padayachee, "Doomsday Forecasts of the AIDS Epidemic" (opinion), *South African Medical Journal* 78 (1990): 503.

29. Sher, "HIV Infection in South Africa, 1982–1988," 317.

30. Schall, Padayachee, and Yach, "The Case for Surveillance in South Africa," 324.

Chapter 2

1. Steve Biko, *Black Consciousness in South Africa*, ed. Millard Arnold (New York: Random House, 1978).

2. "HIV Becomes Prescribed Minimum Benefit," http://www.health24.com/medical/ Condition_centres/777–792–2002–2007,30583.asp (accessed 15 May 2006).

3. Solomon R. Benatar, "Health Care Reform and the Crisis of HIV and AIDS in South Africa," *New England Journal of Medicine* 351 (2004): 81.

4. Nicoli Nattrass, "AIDS, Science and Governance: The Battle over Antiretroviral Therapy in Post-Apartheid South Africa" (19 March 2006), unpublished paper.

5. Virginia van der Vliet, "South Africa Divided against AIDS: A Crisis of Leadership," in Kyle D. Kauffman and David L. Lindauer (eds.), *AIDS and South Africa: The Social Expression of a Pandemic* (New York: Palgrave Macmillan, 2004), 56.

Chapter 3

1. Allister Sparks, *The Mind of South Africa: The Story of the Rise and Fall of Apartheid* (Johannesburg and Cape Town: Ball, 1990), 114–117.

2. Salim S. Abdool Karim, Tandi Zigubu-Page, and Rudewaan Arendse, "Bridging the Gap: Potential for Health Care Partnership between African Traditional Healers and Biomedical Personnel in South Africa," *South African Medical Journal* 84 (Suppl.) (1994): 7–8.

3. Ibid., 2.

Chapter 4

1. O. Shisana, E. Hall, K. R. Maluleke, D. J. Stoker, C. Schwabe, M. Colvin, J. Chauveau, C. Botha, T. Gumede, H. Fomundam, N. Shaikh, T. Rehle, E. Udjo, and D. Grisselquist, "The Impact of HIV/AIDS on the Health Sector: National Survey of Health Personnel, Ambulatory and Hospitalized Patients and Health Facilities" (2003), unpublished report prepared for the South African Department of Health, xiii.

2. Solomon R. Benatar, "Health Care Reform and the Crisis of HIV and AIDS in South Africa," *New England Journal of Medicine* 351 (2004): 81–92.

3. Greg Behrman, *The Invisible People* (New York: Free Press, 2004).

4. Charlene Smith, "Zuma Resists Rape/HIV Studies," *Mail and Guardian*, 21 May 1999, 8.

5. Virginia van der Vliet, "South Africa Divided against AIDS: A Crisis of Leadership," in Kyle D. Kauffman and David L. Lindauer (eds.), *AIDS and South Africa: The Social Expression of a Pandemic* (New York: Palgrave Macmillan, 2004), 58.

6. "Mbeki Stokes Row over Anti-AIDS Drug," *Mail and Guardian*, 31 October 1999, http://www.mg.co.za/articledirect.aspx?articleid=166884&area=%2farchives_online_edit (accessed 18 May 2006).

7. Howard Barrell, "Mbeki Fingers the CIA in AIDS Conspiracy," *Mail and Guardian*, 6 October 2000, 4–5.

8. van der Vliet, "South Africa Divided against AIDS," 59–63.

9. Justin Arenstein and Sizwe samaYende, "Losing Its Grip?" *Mail and Guardian*, 22 March 2002, 13; Nawaal Deane, "Hospital Staff 'Victimised' by Department," *Mail and Guardian*, 16 November 2001, 8.

10. "AIDS Battle Set to Return to Court," *Mail and Guardian*, 15 June 2001, http://www.mg.co.za/articledirect.aspx?area=mg_flat&articleid=153759 (accessed 18 May 2006).

11. Ibid.

12. Drew Forrest, "Behind the Smokescreen," *Mail and Guardian*, 26 October 2001, 25.

13. "Castro Hlongwane, Caravans, Cats, Geese, Foot and Mouth and Statistics: HIV/AIDS and the Struggle for the Humanisation of the African," http://virusmyth.net/aids/data/ancdoc.htm (accessed 19 May 2006).

14. Nicoli Nattrass, "AIDS, Science and Governance: The Battle over Antiretroviral Therapy in Post-Apartheid South Africa" (19 March 2006), unpublished paper; Howard Barrell, "Would the Real AIDS Dissident Please Declare," *Mail and Guardian*, 19 March 2002, 2.

15. "Castro Hlongwane, Caravans, Cats, Geese, Foot and Mouth and Statistics."

16. Ibid.

17. Robert Kirby, "Another Bouquet for Our Tourist Attractions," *Mail and Guardian*, 1 August 2003, http://www.mg.co.za/articledirect.aspx?articleid=25994&area=%2finsight%2finsight_col (accessed 17 May 2006); "Manto's Garlic Won't Stop AIDS," *Mail and Guardian*, 10 November 2003, http://www.mg.co.za/articledirect.aspx?articleid=33071&area=%2fbreaking_news%2fbreaking_news__national%2f (accessed 17 May 2006).

18. "Manuel Denies AIDS Drugs 'Voodoo' Comment," *Mail and Guardian*, 20 March, 2003, http://www.mg.co.za/articledirect.aspx?articleid=17433&area=%2fbreaking_news%2fbreaking_news__national%2f (accessed 18 May 2006).

Chapter 5

1. "Sustainable HIV/AIDS Managed Care a Reality," *South African Medical Journal* 89 (1999): 1140.

2. Ronald Bayer and Gerald Oppenheimer, *AIDS Doctors: Voices from the Epidemic* (New York: Oxford University Press, 2000).

3. J. Anthony, E. J. Coetzee, A. P. Kent, Z. M. van der Spuy, L. A. Denny, C. J. M. Stewart, P. R. de Jong, and H. A. van Coeverden de Groot, "HIV in Pregnancy—A Policy Needed," *South African Medical Journal* 85 (1995): 936.

4. P. T. Matchaba and Z. C. Chapanduka, "Paediatric AIDS—Is Now Not the Right Time to Act?" *South African Medical Journal* 87 (1997): 1343–1345.

5. D. Moodley, J. Moodley, and H. M. Coovadia, "Preventing Perinatal HIV Transmission in Developing Countries—Do We Know Enough?" (letter), *South African Medical Journal* 88 (1998): 431–432; James McIntyre, Glenda Gray, and Saul Johnson, "Paediatric AIDS—Is Now Not the Right Time to Act?" (letter), *South African Medical Journal* 88 (1998): 466–467.

6. Marcia Angell, "The Ethics of Clinical Research in the Third World," *New England Journal of Medicine* 337 (1997): 847–849.

7. Howard Barrell and Stuart Hess, "Zuma Defends AZT Policy," *Mail and Guardian*, 16 October 1998, 12.

8. Mark Lurie, Peter Lurie, Carel IJsselmuiden, and Glenda Gray, "Denying Effective Antiretroviral Drugs to HIV-Positive Pregnant Women: The National Government's Flawed Decision," *South African Medical Journal* 89 (1999): 621–623.

9. Steven Robins, "'Long Live Zackie, Long Live': AIDS Activism, Science and Citizenship after Apartheid," *Journal of Southern African Studies* 30 (2004): 651–672.

10. K. D. Bolton and G. J. Hofmeyr, "Reducing Mother-to-Child Transmission of HIV," *South African Medical Journal* 90 (2000): 322–324.

11. "HIVNET 012: A Phase IIB Trial to Determine the Efficacy of Oral AZT and the Efficacy of Oral Nevirapine for the Prevention of Vertical Transmission of HIV-1 Infection in Pregnant Ugandan Women and Their Neonates," http://www.hptn.org/research_studies/hivnet012.asp (accessed 19 May 2006).

12. Nono Simelela, "Cherry-Picking Is the Luxury of Researchers," *Mail and Guardian*, 28 July 2000, 30.

13. Nawaal Deane, "AIDS: TAC vs State," *Mail and Guardian*, 23 November 2001, 8.

14. "Founding Affidavit in the Matter between Treatment Action Campaign, Haroon Saloojee, Children's Rights Centre and Minister of Health, MECS for Health: High Court of South Africa Transvaal Provincial Division," http://www.tac.org/za/Documents/MTCTCourtCase/ccmfound.txt (accessed 22 November 2002).

15. "Excerpt from Judgment TAC and Others v Minister of Health and Others," http://www.cptech.org/ip/health/sa/sa12142001.html (accessed 18 May 2006).

16. Mark Heywood, "Current Developments, Preventing Mother-to-Child HIV Transmission in South Africa: Background, Strategies and Outcomes of the Treatment Action Campaign Case against the Minister of Health," *South African Journal of Human Rights* 19 (2003): 278–315.

17. Ibid., 295.

18. Jaspreet Kindra, "KZN Premier Presses Ahead," *Mail and Guardian*, 15 January 2002, 7.

19. Belinda Beresford, "KZN Jumps State AIDS Ship," *Mail and Guardian*, 1 March 2002, 8.

20. Heywood, "Current Developments, Preventing Mother-to-Child HIV Transmission in South Africa," 278.

21. Sizwe samaYende and Justin Arenstein, "Mpumalanga Stands Firm on Which Hospitals Can Provide Drugs," *Mail and Guardian*, 22 February 2002, 6; Jaspreet Kindra, "Minister's Nod Is Not Enough," *Mail and Guardian*, 8 February 2002, 8; Justin Arenstein, "Manana Sticks to Her Guns," *Mail and Guardian*, 8 February 2002, 8.

22. Anso Thom, "Shambles at AIDS Baby Treatment Sites," *Mail and Guardian*, 27 June 2003, http://www.mg.co.za/articledirect.aspx?articleid=23159&area=%2finsight%2finsight__comment_and_analysis%2f (accessed 18 May 2006).

23. Deane, "AIDS: TAC vs State," 8.

24. Dan Bortolotti, *Hope in Hell: Inside the World of Doctors without Borders* (Buffalo, N.Y.: Firefly, 2004).

25. Greg Behrman, *The Invisible People* (New York: Free Press, 2004), 141–165.

26. Sidney Kark and Emily Kark, *Promoting Community Health: From Pholela to Jerusalem* (Johannesburg: Witwatersrand University Press, 1999).

27. Bortolotti, *Hope in Hell.*

28. Mark Schoofs, "Anglo American Drops Noted Plan on AIDS Drugs," *Wall Street Journal,* 16 April 2002, A19.

29. Shula Marks, "The Silent Scourge? Silicosis, Respiratory Disease and Gold-Mining in South Africa" (n.d.), unpublished paper.

30. "Anglo to Remedy HIV Workforce," *Mail and Guardian,* 8 May 2001, http://www.mg.co.za/articledirect.aspx?articleid=228694&area=/archives__online_edition (accessed 18 May 2006).

31. Mark Schoofs, "Mining Firm Combats AIDS via Drug Plan," *Wall Street Journal,* 7 May 2001, A3.

32. Schoofs, "Anglo American Drops Noted Plan on AIDS Drugs," A19.

33. Glenda Daniels, "Union Takes Anglo to Task," *Mail and Guardian,* 12 October 2001, http://www.mg.co.za/articledirect.aspx?articleid=217884&area=%2farchives__print_edition%2f (accessed 9 July 2003).

34. Chris Bateman, "Internal Strife over Global AIDS Funds," *South African Medical Journal* 92 (2002): 404.

Chapter 6

1. Nawaal Deane, "TAC to Charge Minister over AIDS Deaths," *Mail and Guardian,* 20 March 2003, 7.

2. "Questions and Answers on TAC's Civil Disobedience Campaign," *Mail and Guardian,* 20 March 2003, 12.

3. Zackie Achmat, "The Long Walk to Civil Disobedience," *Mail and Guardian,* 4 April 2003, 29.

4. Jaspreet Kindra, "Federation May Back TAC," *Mail and Guardian,* 20 March 2003, 11.

5. Nawaal Deane, "Manto Buys Time for AIDS Plan," *Mail and Guardian,* 20 June 2003, 6.

6. Nawaal Deane, "The Devil Is in the Detail," *Mail and Guardian,* 18 July 2003, 6.

7. Government of South Africa, Department of Health, *Operational Plan for Comprehensive HIV and AIDS Care, Management and Treatment for South Africa* (19 November 2003).

8. "Singing the Same Old Tune," *Mail and Guardian,* 27 February 2004, 30.

9. Personal communication, F. Hassan and D. Bosch, AIDS Law Project Monitoring Unit, 20 September 2006.

10. Ibid.

11. Nicoli Nattrass, "Trading Off Income and Health? AIDS and the Disability Grant in South Africa," *Journal of Social Politics* 35 (2005): 3–19.

12. Tom Happold, "Mandela's Eldest Son Dies of AIDS," *Guardian,* 6 January 2005, http://www.guardian.co.uk/aids/story/0,,1384733,00.html (accessed 19 May 2005).

BIOGRAPHICAL NOTES

Quarraisha Abdool Karim was born in Tongaat, South Africa, in 1960. She is an epidemiologist at the Nelson R. Mandela School of Medicine in Durban.

Jamila Aboobaker was born in India in 1945. She is the head of the Department of Dermatology at the Nelson R. Mandela School of Medicine and at the King Edward VIII Hospital in Durban.

Farida Amod was born in South Africa in 1967. She is an internist and a medical microbiologist at the Nelson R. Mandela School of Medicine in Durban.

Caroline Armstrong was born in the United Kingdom in 1967. She is a doctor at the HIV clinic at Grey's Hospital in Pietermaritzburg.

Ann Barnard was born in the United Kingdom in 1969. She is the medical director of Ingwavuma Orphan Care.

Martha Bedelu was born in Ethiopia in 1974. At the time of the interview, she was a doctor treating HIV in a Médecins sans Frontières clinic in Khayelitsha, outside Cape Town.

Linda-Gail Bekker was born in Rhodesia (present-day Zimbabwe) in 1962. She is the medical director of the HIV clinic at Guguletu, outside Cape Town, and a principal investigator at the Desmond Tutu HIV Centre at the University of Cape Town.

Ramesh Laloo Bhoola was born in Durban, South Africa, in 1943. A general practitioner with an interest in gastroenterology, he is in private practice.

Raziya Bobat was born in Durban, South Africa, in 1954. She is a specialist in the Department of Pediatrics and Child Health at the Nelson R. Mandela School of Medicine and at the King Edward VIII Hospital in Durban.

Mariëtte Botes was born in South Africa in 1966. She is a hospital-based general practitioner who specializes in HIV in Pretoria.

Brian Brink was born in Johannesburg, South Africa, in 1952. A doctor, he is the Senior Vice President for health at Anglo American South Africa.

Edwin Cameron was born in Pretoria, South Africa, in 1953. He is a justice on the Supreme Court of Appeal, South Africa.

Laura Campbell was born in Northern Ireland in 1962. A doctor working in Port Shepstone, she has a special interest in HIV palliative care.

Salome Charalambous was born in the North West Province of South Africa in 1973. A doctor, she works for the Aurum Institute for Health Research, which is associated with the Anglo American Corporation.

Gavin Churchyard was born in Northern Rhodesia (present-day Zambia) in 1958. An internist and epidemiologist, he directs the Aurum Institute for Health Research, which is associated with the Anglo American Corporation.

Ashraf Coovadia was born in Zambia in 1965. He is a specialist in pediatrics at Coronation Women and Children's Hospital in Johannesburg.

Hoosen "Jerry" Coovadia was born in South Africa in 1941. He is a specialist in pediatrics and a professor of HIV/AIDS research at the Nelson R. Mandela School of Medicine in Durban.

Felicity Cope was born in Rhodesia (present-day Zimbabwe) in 1944. She was an infection control nurse at Groote Schuur and then Somerset hospitals.

Mark Cotton was born in Cape Town, South Africa, in 1956. He is a physician in the Department of Pediatrics and Child Health at Tygerberg Children's Hospital in Cape Town.

Jeanne Dixon was born in Sterkstroom, South Africa, in 1943. She is a retired nurse who started the HIV/AIDS program at Grey's Hospital in Pietermaritzburg.

François Eksteen was born in Upington, South Africa. He is an internal medicine specialist and runs a pediatric HIV/AIDS clinic at the Church of Scotland Hospital in Tugela Ferry in KwaZulu-Natal.

Clive Evian was born in South Africa in 1951. He is a community health specialist who heads an HIV consulting firm.

Elizabeth Fielder was born in the United Kingdom in 1938. She is a nurse and senior trials manager at the Desmond Tutu HIV Centre at the University of Cape Town.

Bernhard Gaede was born in Roodepoort, South Africa, in 1966. He is a doctor at Emmaus Hospital in Winterton in KwaZulu-Natal.

Eric Goemaere was born in Belgium in 1954. A doctor, he is head of mission for Médecins sans Frontières, South Africa, and directs its AIDS work at Khayelitsha, outside Cape Town.

Glenda Gray was born in Boksburg, South Africa, in 1962. She is a pediatrician and director of the Perinatal HIV Research Unit at Chris Hani Baragwanath Hospital in Johannesburg.

Ashraf Grimwood was born in South Africa in 1958. A doctor, he heads a network of clinics funded by the British charity ARK (Absolute Return for Kids) and has a private practice in Cape Town.

Musa Gumede was born in South Africa in 1968. A doctor, he has a private practice in Durban.

Jane Hampton was born in Rhodesia (present-day Zimbabwe) in 1955. She is a doctor at McCord Hospital's Sinikithemba HIV/AIDS Care Center in Durban.

Mark Heywood was born in Nigeria in 1964. He is a human rights activist who works with the AIDS Law Project and the Treatment Action Campaign.

Helga Holst was born in Canada in 1952. She is the medical superintendent of McCord Hospital in Durban.

David Johnson was born in South Africa in 1962. A family practitioner, he has a private practice in Johannesburg.

Saul Johnson was born in Johannesburg, South Africa, in 1965. A pediatrician, he is the director of Health and Development Africa, a health consulting company.

Alan Karstaedt was born in South Africa in 1953. A doctor, he directs the adult HIV/AIDS clinic at Chris Hani–Baragwanath Hospital in Johannesburg.

Paul Kocheleff was born in Belgium in 1937. An internist and cardiologist, he works with the HIV clinics at Edendale and Grey's hospitals in Pietermaritzburg.

Veliswa Labatala was born in Guguletu, South Africa, in 1974. She is a nurse working in Médecins sans Frontières' rape clinic in Khayelitsha, outside Cape Town.

Umesh Lalloo was born in South Africa in 1956. A pulmonologist, he is head of the Department of Medicine at the Nelson R. Mandela School of Medicine and at King Edward VIII Hospital in Durban.

Leon Levin was born in Benoni, South Africa, in 1963. A pediatrician, formerly at Johannesburg Hospital, he has a private practice.

Gary Maartens was born in South Africa in 1956. He is an internist specializing in infectious disease at Groote Schuur Hospital in Cape Town.

Themba Mabaso was born in Durban, South Africa, in 1963. A doctor, he has a private practice in Durban.

Gabi Mbanjwa was born in South Africa in 1961. She is a nurse specializing in HIV/AIDS at King Edward VIII Hospital in Durban.

James McIntyre was born in Rhodesia (present-day Zimbabwe) in 1956. A specialist in obstetrics and gynecology, he directs the Perinatal HIV Research Unit at Chris Hani–Baragwanath Hospital in Johannesburg.

Neil McKerrow was born in Welkom, South Africa, in 1956. He is a pediatrician and head of the pediatric departments at Grey's and Northdale hospitals in Pietermaritzburg.

Tammy Meyers was born in Johannesburg, South Africa, in 1961. She is head of the pediatric AIDS clinic at Chris Hani Baragwanath Hospital in Johannesburg.

Steven Miller was born in South Africa in 1954. He is a private practitioner in Johannesburg.

Clarence Mini was born in East London, South Africa, in 1951. A doctor, he works with hospice patients and chairs the board of the National Association of People Living with HIV/AIDS (NAPWA).

Aresh Misra was born in South Africa in 1968. A family practitioner, he has a private practice in Durban.

May Mkhize was born in the Eastern Transvaal (present-day Mpumalanga) in South Africa in 1956. A doctor, she oversees an HIV clinic in Vulindlela in KwaZulu-Natal.

Kathryn Mngadi was born in Durban, South Africa, in 1964. A doctor, at the time of the interview she headed AngloGold's HIV wellness clinic in Orkney in the North West Province.

Tony Moll was born in Rhodesia (present-day Zimbabwe) in 1954. A doctor, he directs AIDS services at the Church of Scotland Hospital in Tugela Ferry in KwaZulu-Natal.

Yunus Moosa was born in 1962. He is head of infectious disease at King Edward VIII Hospital in Durban.

Anisa Mosam was born in Durban, South Africa, in 1968. She is a dermatologist at King Edward VIII Hospital in Durban.

Eula Mothibi was born in Kimberley, South Africa, in 1966. She is a hospital-based internist who has worked in Cape Town and was responsible for the antiretroviral rollout in Northern Cape Province.

Lulu Mtwisha was born in Transkei, South Africa, in 1940. A nurse, she trains and coordinates therapeutic counselors for the Desmond Tutu HIV Centre at the University of Cape Town.

James Muller was born in Cape Town, South Africa, in 1949. He heads the Department of Medicine of the Pietermaritzburg Metropolitan Hospital Complex.

Kogie Naidoo was born in Durban, South Africa, in 1969. She is a pediatrician at King Edward VIII Hospital and a project director for the Centre for the AIDS Programme of Research in South Africa at the Nelson R. Mandela School of Medicine in Durban.

Dalu Ndiweni was born in Rhodesia (present-day Zimbabwe) in 1957. A pediatrician, he heads the pediatric AIDS clinic at Johannesburg Hospital.

Lucky Ndokweni was born in South Africa in 1958. He is a doctor in private practice in Durban.

Nomangesi Judith "Pinky" Ngcakani was born in the Eastern Cape Province of South Africa in 1969. A doctor, she is in private practice in Durban.

Paul Nijs was born in Belgium in 1948. A doctor, he heads Edendale Hospital's adult AIDS clinics in Pietermaritzburg.

Nontuthuzelo Ntwana was born in Transkei (present-day Eastern Cape), South Africa, in 1966. She is a nurse at Médecins sans Frontières' general medicine clinic in Khayelitsha, outside Cape Town.

Liesl Page-Shipp was born in Johannesburg, South Africa, in 1969. A doctor, at the time of the interview she worked for the Aurum Institute for Health Research, which is associated with the Anglo American Corporation.

Hermann Reuter was born in Namibia in 1968. A doctor, he is the director of the Médecins sans Frontières' Lusikisiki HIV program in the Eastern Cape Province.

Sue Roberts was born in Ficksburg, South Africa. She is an infection control nurse at Helen Joseph Hospital in Johannesburg.

Andrew Ross was born in the United Kingdom in 1962. He is a doctor at St. Mary's Hospital and works with the Department of Rural Health at the Nelson R. Mandela School of Medicine in Durban.

Paul Roux was born in South Africa in 1950. He is a pediatrician and head of pediatric HIV/AIDS services at Groote Schuur Hospital in Cape Town.

Haroon Saloojee was born in Johannesburg, South Africa, in 1961. A neonatologist at Chris Hani–Baragwanath Hospital at the time of the interview, he is now the head of the Division of Community Pediatrics in the Department of Pediatrics and Child Health at the University of Witwatersrand in Johannesburg.

Ian Sanne was born in South Africa in 1967. An internist, he is head of the Clinical HIV Research Unit at the University of Witwatersrand in Johannesburg.

Hannah Mothshedisi Sebitloane was born in the North West Province of South Africa in 1967. She is a doctor specializing in obstetrics and gynecology at the Nelson R. Mandela School of Medicine and at King Edward VIII Hospital in Durban.

Margaret Shangase was born in South Africa in 1942. She is a retired nurse who served as AIDS coordinator for the HIV/AIDS clinic at Edendale Hospital in Pietermaritzburg and later as a regional director for AIDS services in KwaZulu-Natal.

Ruben Sher was born in South Africa in 1929. An infectious disease specialist, he is the director of HIVCare International.

Dennis Sifris was born in Johannesburg, South Africa, in 1945. A general practitioner, he has a private practice in Johannesburg.

David Spencer was born in South Africa in 1950. An internist with training in infectious disease, he has a private practice in Johannesburg.

Henry Sunpath was born in Durban, South Africa, in 1961. A doctor, he directs clinical services at McCord Hospital's Sinikithemba HIV/AIDS Care Center.

Bongani Thembela was born in KwaZulu-Natal in South Africa in 1958. An internist, he works in the King Edward VIII Hospital's Department of General Medicine in Durban.

Robin Wood was born in the United Kingdom in 1948. A doctor, he is a principal investigator at the Desmond Tutu HIV Centre at the University of Cape Town.

INDEX OF INDIVIDUALS INTERVIEWED

INDEX